FAT BIRTH

MICHELLE MAYEFSKE

Book Cover Design by Charlotte Thomson-Morley
Print Book and E-book Interior Design by Ashley Santoro
Editing by Amber Hatch and Salt & Sage Books
Author Photography by Natalja Vorozcova

ISBN 978-1-7372091-0-2

Significant discounts for bulk sales are available.
Please contact Michelle at www.fatandpregnant.com

Table of Contents

Dedication:
For Aidan, Niamh, William, Graham and Iris—my little loves x

Introduction:

THE CONCEPTION OF FAT BIRTH

I was catapulted into the world of birth activism unintentionally. My great -grandmother was not a midwife nor was anyone in my family or group of friends passionate about birth. Like most people, birth was not on my radar until I found myself pregnant—though my journey to parenthood was unlike most. Following a brief rebound relationship, fueled by irresponsibility and a complete disregard for the effectiveness of birth control, I found myself pregnant unexpectedly at the age of sixteen. With no unbiased guide, real life experience or internal wisdom to rely upon, I had little knowledge to help me navigate the sheer magnitude of pregnancy. The childbirth education I received from my teen parent classes was very surface-level and lacked even a whiff of what self advocacy was or why it might be necessary. While I imagined my birth being a calm, low-intervention experience, it quickly turned into something else on the day.

Like many first-time moms, my labor started spontaneously and was slowly progressing in a hospital setting. Both my baby and I were doing well, however, my nurses strongly suggested Pitocin to speed up the labor process. I was not given the proper information regarding potential side effects, and I became frightened when things started spinning out of control. The rest of my son's birth involved hyperstimulation of my uterus, narcotic pain relief, memory loss and being demanded to fight against the *incredible* urge to push until an obstetrician walked into the room. While my pregnancy ended with the birth of a healthy baby boy, I was left feeling confused, overwhelmed and shell-shocked… and no one cared.

I accepted the complete railroading of my birth experience because I simply did not know anything different. The majority of what I had seen on television were dramatic, frantic, panicked depictions of birth. I did my best to put my negative birth experience behind me and spent the next five years both raising and growing up alongside my son, Aidan. I finished high school and completed my college degree thanks to the loving support of both my parents. And let me tell you—I was not an easy person to love or support back then.

I had a major psychological growth spurt in my early twenties when I met the Irish man of my dreams. Anthony and I were married in 2009 and we moved to Ireland shortly after. Following more than two years of dealing with the stress of trying to conceive, I saw the double pink lines of a positive pregnancy-test in 2011.

Navigating maternity care in a country that still felt new to me was overwhelming. Thanks to some online forums, I came across an expecting mom in Ireland who was preparing for her home birth. One online search for "home birth Ireland" led to a flood of information and resources that were both refreshing and infuriating. The more I learned, the more I was able to reflect on my first birth experience and envision how birth could be different—and better!

I continued exploring my options and ultimately decided that a home birth felt like the best option for our family. Once I submerged myself within Ireland's home birth community, I began noticing the obvious barriers to Ireland's national health service. The criteria that impacted me directly were the body mass index (BMI) specifications. Having a BMI over thirty-five put a fat person like me in a "grey area," meaning I would need the approval of a doctor to go ahead with my plans. This was my first brushing with weight stigma within maternity culture, and it made me feel very shameful about my body. The BMI guidelines certainly made me wonder how my birth options could be limited simply because of my size.

Despite these guidelines, I decided to push on and finally worked up enough courage to call a community midwife. I spoke openly to her and peeled back many layers of vulnerability when I told her my biggest fear—that my weight might "risk me out" of the home birth service. I further disclosed my exact BMI and instead of being met with compassion or support, I heard the cold, callous response, "Oh wow, *you are big!*" After this humiliating experience, I lost all hope in finding anyone who would see me as more than a number on the scale.

After a whirlwind of change, our family moved to Wisconsin, USA (where I am originally from) when I was five months pregnant and when Aidan was almost eight years old. With a lack of midwifery options and funds, Anthony and I decided a home birth was not on the cards for us. After much discussion, we compromised and continued planning for a hospital birth with the support of a doula. Jade was the first person who truly believed in my fat body's ability to birth. Anthony and I met with her multiple times throughout my pregnancy to go over birth preferences, what to expect in the hospital and how to best prepare for a more positive experience. As a result, my daughter's birth was much more positive and it sparked in me a passion for birth rights that has never faded.

Over the next six years I went on to birth two more babies at home and trained to become a birth doula and childbirth educator. I learned more during each pregnancy and became increasingly passionate about defending the birth rights of others. While this aspect of my identity continued to develop, the road to body neutrality and fat activism—which ultimately led to the writing of this book—took much longer.

Like so many people, my childhood was fraught with fatphobia and body shame. It is particularly painful to look back on because of the enormous hatred I held for the body I was born into. That hatred was also continuously fueled by someone I love very much but who is also the most fatphobic person I know, my mother. Just like today, in the 1980s and 1990s, fat shaming was seen as acceptable by society at large. It was also a toxic thread woven into the fabric of my otherwise loving family home.

Fatphobia became a pervasive aspect of my life, beginning at six months old. My mother had taken me to a standard wellness check with our family doctor. At this appointment my doctor evaluated my little, soft baby body, took out his imaginary crystal ball and told my mother that I was doomed to struggle with my weight for the rest of my life. As a fatphobic parent who could imagine nothing worse than raising a fat child, alarm bells began sounding in my mother's brain. She went on to do everything in her power to prevent my predicted fatness, while simultaneously and unintentionally creating a life filled with body shame and disordered eating. Throughout my entire childhood food was hidden from me and I was scolded for eating the wrong things or sneaking food. Some of my earliest childhood memories include being told repeatedly to, "Stop sticking out your belly," and going to Weight Watchers meetings. My mother and I regularly walked across the carpeted floors of the stale-smelling room and found a place to sit amongst the semicircle of chairs, ready for the latest motivation for dieters.

By the time I was eleven years old, my mother—who was clearly unhappy with her own body size—had me start tracking what I ate using a points system along with her. Although she may have thought her actions were good, my mom was oblivious to the cascade of disordered eating she had initiated me into. The more I continue to speak with people who were fat or "chubby" as children, the more I realize my childhood experience is not unique. So many people have been encouraged to diet or "watch what they ate" as kids.

From the age of eleven and into my teen years, I was constantly dieting, whether I recognized it as such or not. I began to view my body's hunger cues and appetite as problems that needed to be solved, or at least ignored. By fourteen, I was no longer following any diet plan or points system. I had one goal—eat as little as possible, and it worked. I was suffering from atypical anorexia—engaging in all of the behaviors associated with the illness, although technically my BMI was not "low enough" for a formal diagnosis at the time. I continued severe disordered eating until I got pregnant at sixteen.

Once I allowed myself to eat during my first pregnancy, I experienced a phenomenon described by Evelyn Tribole and Elyse Resch, as "rebound eating."[1] I temporarily dropped all food rules and gave myself permission to eat—and did I ever! I gained over eighty pounds during the remainder of my pregnancy, securely landing myself into a high BMI category where I would inevitably stay.

My issues with body image and disordered eating continued throughout my adult life and played into my subsequent three pregnancies—which spanned over fourteen years. I was always monitoring my weight, stepping on the scale every morning and checking my "progress." I never questioned how my disordered methods were impacting my physical and mental health, even during pregnancy. Following all four of my births, my continued obsession with the thin ideal meant postpartum life was bogged down by diet-focused thoughts. After my youngest child was born in 2017, I knew something needed to change.

One year postpartum, I came across an intuitive eating coach online, named Jen. She began guiding me through steps toward body neutrality and intuitive eating via a series of weekly video consultations. I found myself buying all the anti-diet, intuitive eating and body positive books I could get my hands on. My mind was being opened to ideas that I had never thought possible. I began to learn body respect and how to appreciate all of the things my body *could do*—like grow and birth four amazing humans. This is also when I started exploring all of the ways diet culture and weight discrimination have caused harm to people of size, including those who are pregnant.

It is no surprise that I would marry my two biggest passions, birth advocacy and fat activism. When I began searching for resources specifically related to plus size pregnancy, what I found was an incredible void. Of the limited content available, the vast majority focused primarily on risks, complications and worst-case scenarios. It is no wonder so many people of size have resigned themselves to believing that their body is destined to be a host of problems. That has been the most prevalent narrative of fatness—as an illness and disorder.

In 2019, I started the Instagram account @fat.and.pregnant to create a fat positive platform where I could share size-friendly information with fat people all over the world. I also sought to actively challenge the harmful, fatphobic ways people approach plus size birth. When I conceived my fifth baby in the fall of 2019, I chose to share my firsthand experiences of being fat and pregnant on a daily basis. I was prepared for some communication from my followers, however, I was not prepared for the dozens of messages I would receive every day. Many of the messages were thank-yous, however, most were examples of provider weight stigma and people looking for support and information that they *were not finding anywhere else*. I cannot possibly share all of the messages but these are some very common themes shared by self-identifying fat folks:

- Being told they could not possibly give birth vaginally
- Persistent fat shaming remarks at prenatal visits
- Being advised to lose weight or "maintain their weight" throughout pregnancy
- Providers telling them they have to do something: be weighed, take blood thinners, get an epidural in early labor and more. What in reality are all options, were presented as mandatory
- Being labeled as a "high-risk" pregnancy with the guarantee that something would go wrong

Both the Fat and Pregnant website and *Fat Birth* book have been created to help share the knowledge and information so desperately needed within the fat community. Both of these resources advocate for information sharing that is unbiased, holistic and centered around the individual needs of plus size people—with the absence of weight bias, of course. *Fat Birth* has been written within an anti-diet framework. This means that the diversity of body shapes and sizes is respected within these pages. Being fat is not viewed as a problem nor something that needs to be "fixed." This also means that one's body size is not seen as indicative of their state of health, which is discussed more in Chapter One. I understand that these ideas may feel new and radical for some people and that's okay. At its core, the *Fat Birth* book believes that all bodies are seen as worthy of dignified and compassionate maternity care, no matter their size or health status. As such, you will not read any suggestions for dieting, weight loss or changing your body in any way. You will learn ways to navigate common challenges experienced during plus size pregnancy and gain practical tools so you are better able to advocate for yourself and ensure your best interests are always at the center of your care. I hope this book is a springboard for you to explore these topics, whether you are currently trying to conceive, are pregnant or you support others during these stages of life.

While writing this book, I was very aware of not wanting to sound like an "angry fat woman"—but here's the truth—*I am an angry fat woman* who wants other fat people to know that they deserve better. Fat people deserve to be treated with dignity and respect. My passion for this topic will shine through my writing. I have also included some hard truths and I hope as a reader you will understand why. Some people, usually birth workers of some kind, may believe they are "protecting mothers" by denying them the information they truly need, because the reality may be viewed as "too harsh" or intense. I share it all. Leaving out information and skirting around tough subjects only promotes further ignorance and harm.

Fat Birth is laid out in two sections, with the first packed full of information to help you prepare for your best birth. Like any resource, not everything found in these pages will apply to you. You are the only expert on your body and your life, so take away what feels right and leave the rest. The second section contains a rich collection of positive birth stories submitted by plus size parents from across the globe. Every individual's birth story is personal to them and I hope you appreciate the vulnerability that comes with sharing these intimate memories. Make sure you have a tissue handy!

You will close the covers of *Fat Birth* knowing the following:

- You are worthy of a joyful pregnancy.
- Your weight does not limit what your amazing, pregnant body is capable of .
- That all types of birth can be experienced in a positive way.

Author's Notes

There are many words that are used to refer to people living in bigger bodies. These include but are not limited to: plus size, fat, person of size, overweight, obese and more. Many fat activists have worked tirelessly to reclaim and strip away the stigma and biases associated with the word "fat" which has historically been used to bully and abuse others.

Within this text I will treat the word fat as a non-medical, neutral descriptor of body size. I will not use the words "overweight" and "obese" because both imply fatness is an illness or outside of a socially constructed norm.

Throughout the book I refer to pregnant and birthing individuals in multiple ways: women, woman, mother, parent, birthing person, pregnant person, expecting parent and more. I understand and acknowledge that not all pregnant and birthing people identify as female. This book is intended for any person looking for information regarding fat pregnancy and birth.

This book is not meant to advocate for any particular way of giving birth. The information provided is not intended to replace any medical advice given to you by your midwife, obstetrician or other medical provider. The author and publisher disclaim any liability directly or indirectly from the use of the materials within this text.

Chapter One:

THE STORY WE ARE TOLD

"I feel like every appointment has been a battle since week twelve. All my bloodwork and tests come back normal but I'm constantly having to fight against being induced 'because of my size.' I'm holding my ground but it is getting exhausting. Please tell me there's another way."

Crystal had done what most people do once they discover they are pregnant—she booked an appointment with her doctor to confirm her pregnancy and began looking for information and prenatal resources online. Sadly, what Crystal kept coming in contact with is the "one story" of fat pregnancy, which I call the *"fearful fat"* narrative. As a plus size expecting parent, she was looking for helpful tips, a community of support and ways to prepare for a positive pregnancy and birth. What she heard and read instead was a collection of fat shaming, worst-case scenarios and risk-based information. Not only did the excitement surrounding her pregnancy feel deflated, but she had also become increasingly fearful for both herself and her baby. She reached out to me for unbiased support and information that would help her feel more confident and in control of her experience.

We live during a time and within a culture which seems to only share a single narrative of fat pregnancy—it is portrayed as risky, challenging, dangerous, complicated and prone to intervention. Many parents may be led to believe they are certainly more likely, if not guaranteed, to develop health issues throughout pregnancy and their birth will be anything but straight forward. Assumptions about their lifestyle, strength and ability are common, with most of their maternity care revolving around their weight. In many cases fat pregnancy and birth are automatically viewed as "high-risk," and as such, need to be monitored, managed and controlled appropriately. Expecting parents may be told that not only have they been irresponsible with their own health, but now their fatness may have negative consequences for their baby. Passivity is encouraged, with a "doctor knows best" approach being standard with assumed compliance. *This is just the way pregnancy is for fat folks.* This story is internalized and carried by fat people everywhere, who believe it is all they deserve, trapped within the pages of these harmful stereotypes.

"It's not if you will develop a problem, but when."

Chimamanda Ngozi Adichie explains the dangers behind the sharing of a single story such as this: "The single story creates stereotypes and the problem with stereotypes is not that they are untrue but that they are incomplete. They make one story become the only story."[1]

In the case of fat pregnancy, these stereotypes have led to general pathologization, or the treating of all fat pregnancies as an illness that must be monitored and managed with an interventionist approach. When we look at the lived experiences of those who are fat and pregnant, we need to consider whose stories we hear and who the storytellers are. Are we listening to fat folks themselves or is someone else sharing and controlling this *fearful fat* narrative? If it is someone else, do they have something to gain by maintaining this story?

Chimamanda Ngozi Adichie goes on to explain the issue of power within single story telling—"Power is the ability not only to tell the story of another person but to make it the definitive story of that person," ensuring the story is told over and over.[1] This is evidenced when the same grim story of plus size pregnancy is predominantly depicted and reinforced within the media, by those we love and in the very offices we access for prenatal care. When fatness is portrayed as something we need to fear, it becomes easier for others to exert power and attempt to control fat bodies during pregnancy and birth. When the focus of this narrative is solely on risks, potential challenges and the medicalization of fat bodies, the incredible experience of pregnancy is flattened and ignored. Instead of promoting confidence and strength during birth, the agency of people of size is lost as they fearfully await the negative outcomes they were warned about all along.

In order to understand this single story and how it has prevailed for so long, we must take a step back and look at the three things that underpin this fatphobic narrative: diet culture, weight stigma and BMI.

DIET CULTURE

Diet culture is the belief system that teaches us that both our self worth and abilities are linked directly to our physical appearance. It promotes thinness at all costs, regardless of the impacts to our physical and emotional health. It thrives on our ability to compare ourselves to one another and make judgements based on what we see. It upholds and is fueled by the predominant belief that fat is the worst thing we could possibly be. Diet culture is behind the many stereotypes associated with being fat and it benefits from these stereotypes going unquestioned. Fat means laziness. Fat means a lack of willpower, self control and self respect. It is viewed as shameful, ugly and a symptom of not taking care of oneself. Diet culture capitalizes on these messages we constantly receive, allowing businesses to make promises that if we try hard enough and spend enough time and money, that we too can transform ourselves into the ideal, the "ideal" being thin. This standard of beauty actively aims to reduce body diversity and has contributed to people becoming increasingly fearful of fatness.

Fatphobia can be described in many ways but is often depicted as the fear of being around fat people, being or becoming fat. Fatphobia impacts people's behavior, their thoughts and how they treat those living in bigger bodies.

Diet culture ensures that the weight loss and beauty industries make billions of dollars every year as they try to shape our expectations about what our bodies should and should not look like. These culturally-created narrow beauty standards of femininity are also applied to pregnancy and postpartum. We are marketed "solutions" to our perceived body problems that are both created and sold by the beauty and weight loss industries, ensuring they remain profitable. This body preoccupation so many of us have felt during our lifetime is the direct result of industry exploitation. It is the reason we buy products and join slimming clubs that promise to "fix" our perceived imperfections, including our body size. Such body worries promote disordered eating in an effort to shed pounds, often done when people are trying to conceive, during pregnancy and postpartum.

The pressure to be thin is upheld during these life stages and can prove harmful for both expecting parents and their babies. Both diet culture and the industries who benefit from body shame make a profit as they maintain the single narrative that fat bodies are a problem that need to be fixed. If bigger bodies cannot be fixed, at the very least, they must be managed and blamed for not adhering to the status quo. This is directly seen within the *fearful fat* narrative.

WEIGHT STIGMA

We cannot escape the reality that many people believe being fat and pregnant is wrong or irresponsible—some even call it criminal.[2] These people, including medical professionals, are influenced by the same toxic cultural attitudes promoted by diet culture. They often believe fat bodies are broken, that weight is the best indicator of health and that our bodies, and especially our babies, need to be "rescued" by our fatness. Society in general assigns moral value to those seen as "looking after themselves" and if you are fat and pregnant, it is assumed that clearly you are not doing so. Once you investigate the lies we are told which contribute to the *fearful fat* pregnancy story, you can choose to stop believing them.

Our fatphobic society, and medical system work incredibly hard to share and promote the *fearful fat* narrative in an effort to further convince us that any diagnosis or complication during pregnancy *must* be the result of our defective fat bodies. The *reality,* however, is that there is no pregnancy complication that is solely attributed to people of size. *Anyone* can experience the "big three" pregnancy health issues that are often peddled as complications primarily associated with fatness: gestational diabetes, gestational hypertension and preeclampsia. When you learn the truth about these health issues and the *absolute risk* of developing them, you begin to realize that fear does not have to be the foundation of your experience—there is another way. It is both weight bias and weight stigma which contribute to the culture of fear surrounding pregnancy in a bigger body.

Weight stigma is the social disapproval and discrimination targeted at others due to their weight and size. It the last form of discrimination that is seen as socially acceptable and it is the most common form of stigma seen within the medical community. Weight stigma is the direct result of weight bias, sometimes called anti-fat bias, which is the negative beliefs and opinions people have associated with weight. Every individual may have explicit and/or implicit weight, which have developed over time. Explicit bias is when someone is aware of the prejudices and attitudes they have regarding a person or group of people. An implicit bias is when a person has unconscious attitudes, beliefs or stereotypes regarding a group of people. Implicit bias affects a person's behavior and may go against the values that a person consciously holds, which can also be challenging to accept.

Most people accept that weight bias exists, however, they have trouble swallowing how prevalent it is and how it translates to the medical community. One study found that 67% of almost 5,000 medical students in the United States exhibited an explicit bias whose "...attitudes were more negative toward ob[*]se people than toward racial minorities, gays, lesbians, and poor people."[3] Those with implicit and explicit anti-fat bias were more likely to be male, with a lower BMI, from an affluent family background and non-Black. I cannot be the only person not surprised that privileged, thin white guys tend to be more biased. Another study aimed to assess the level of weight bias of trainee dieticians, nutritionists, nurses and doctors within the UK highlighted this stark reality. These professionals were selected because they would be the medics who will have the most direct contact with a people of size and whose role it is to help them. Alarmingly, the study found that 98.6% of this next generation of healthcare workers possess "unacceptable levels of weight bias."[4] Dr Gregory Dodell, an endocrinologist in the United States, has publicly shared his thoughts on why we see students with such high levels of bias—"Fatphobia is ingrained from the earliest stages of medical training. It is a top down problem,"[5] and one whose effects will impact countless fat people just trying to access respectful medical care. These medical students will begin their careers with already firmly planted negative attitudes and stereotypes towards fat people.

The role of healthcare providers is to improve their patient's health, longevity and quality of life through respectful, individualized care—and weight bias gets in the way of this! When weight bias presents within the medical community, it is associated with poorer health outcomes, delayed diagnoses amongst fat folks, hormone dysregulation, healthcare avoidance, mistreatment within clinical settings and profound negative effects on mental health.[6]

People who are mistreated as a result of anti-fat bias are more likely to experience prolonged levels of stress and develop a mistrust of doctors.[7]

People are subjected to weight biased information every single day, both inside and outside of the healthcare setting. It impacts how people feel, their sense of worthiness and value as fat and pregnant people. It is also important to note that weight stigma occurs along a spectrum, so not all people of size will experience it the same way. Someone who wears a size thirty may experience weight stigma completely differently from someone who identifies as a "small fat," at a size eighteen. We must recognize that all forms of weight stigma are harmful and that they contribute to the *fearful fat* story of pregnancy. This story shapes our perceptions, our beliefs and our expectations of pregnancy. When it is influenced so heavily by weight stigma, we must consider the negative implications it has on the experience of becoming new parents.

Weight stigma is particularly pervasive within the medical community, and maternity care is no exception. It impacts the way maternity care is provided, including: common testing, birth options, decision-making, experiences of coercion, intervention rates and more. Weight stigma lurks in places we would not expect and it has the potential to hurt moms and babies. When you understand the *fearful fat* story of pregnancy, you recognize how it is influenced by weight stigma and the impact this may have on the care you receive. You accept that you may need to advocate for yourself when you come face-to-face with a health system that discriminates against people based solely on their size.

It is not fair or acceptable that fat folks have to do this additional work. People of size should not have to use their energy having difficult conversations and setting boundaries with providers who are weight biased. Weight stigma has no place in maternity care, but the reality is that it *does* exist and you have the ability to learn how to navigate this imperfect system. These are some examples of weight stigma and how the *fearful fat* pregnancy story may present itself during maternity care:

- A medical provider makes assumptions about someone's eating habits and level of activity, reminding them, "You're not eating for two." This is often fueled by the stereotype that fat people must not eat well and are lazy.
- An expecting parent is told they must be tested for gestational diabetes repeatedly during pregnancy—beyond the standard two tests, which both came back normal. Again, this is fueled by assumptions, including the idea that all fat people will develop gestational diabetes.
- Someone is advised to lose weight during pregnancy, "for the sake of

their baby."

- A weight biased provider believes fat people are "too big" to birth their babies vaginally. They tell parents of size that a cesarean will be the best option for them with no room for discussion.
- An expecting parent is told, "All big moms make big babies," so an induction is suggested at thirty-eight weeks of pregnancy, despite this not being evidence-based practice.
- A provider equates fatness with weakness, so they do not believe people of size have the strength to birth their babies vaginally. They routinely "allow" twenty minutes of active pushing (which is a ridiculously short amount of time), before they decide to, "just help baby a little," by performing an episiotomy (incision in the perineum) and vacuum-assisted delivery that may not have been necessary.

Weight stigma is often the reason why many fat people feel that a joyful pregnancy and birth is not a possibility for them. People of size, and the majority of expecting parents for that matter, have somehow come to accept that birth is inherently unpleasant, degrading, violating and even traumatic—"Leave your dignity at the door," being uttered to expecting parents who nod in approval. We have also accepted that this type of experience is all we deserve as fat people—"I brought this on myself because of my size." We need to stop tolerating subpar care that pathologizes fatness and demand care that is compassionate, holistic and individualized to our own needs.

BMI

BMI is bullshit. In order to understand why BMI, the body mass index, is an arbitrary number that literally says nothing about *your individual health*, we must first look at the history of this flawed statistic. BMI was originally called the Quetelet Index, named after its Belgian creator, Lambert Adolphe Quetelet. Quetelet was a mathematician, astronomer and sociologist. He was not a doctor nor did he study any form of medicine. Quetelet was known most notably from his sociological work in which he identified the characteristics of "the average man." The Quetelet Index was in part created in the early to mid-1800's because it was a quick and easy way to find the mean weight of a population, which Quetelet believed was also its ideal. His simple formula created this "ideal" for "the average (white) man," which would later be used to scientifically justify eugenics, including the sterilization of large populations.

The Quetelet Index and the BMI we use today are calculated by taking a person's weight (in kilograms) and dividing it by their height squared. It is important to note that the subjects who were studied during the creation of the Quetelet Index were all white males from France and Scotland. Quetelet himself was clear that this measurement was never intended to be applied to individuals as an indicator of health, body fat or build. It was designed to measure entire populations for statistical purposes only.

In 1985, the United States National Instiutes of Health (NIH) adopted the practice that weight classification should be directly linked with BMI. A National Institutes of Health Consensus Development Conference Statement read that it "recommends that physicians adopt this measure"[8] and with that, the flawed BMI statistic meant only for population analysis became enshrined in US public policy. It has since become the norm within physicians' offices everywhere, with many people accepting BMI as a simple truth and a direct measure of size and health.

BMI is also used today for other purposes, including to justify higher premiums for both health insurance and life insurance policies. It has become universally relied upon as an indicator of health with no solid foundations showing it is actually linked to health. BMI is in part problematic because it does not consider other factors which impact weight and overall health, including: genetics, behaviors, environment, education level, income level, age, sex, access to healthcare, trauma and the differences between fat, muscle and bone density. Because BMI is a measure that was created by white people, for white people, it is naturally racist in its origins, as it does not account for any racial differences. This has led to the misclassification of People of Color and continued negative health implications.

Further, the body mass index has proven to be one of the most effective ways to oppress fat people and maintain the narrative that fatness equals badness. It has contributed to the *fearful fat* pregnancy narrative by promoting feelings of shame and anxiety regarding body size. It has upheld the perception that the primary indicator of health is weight, although we now know that there are many lifestyle and behavioral choices which impact our overall wellbeing. This flawed statistic categorizes people into "normal" and "abnormal," which automatically creates a category of "other," leading to continued weight discrimination. If you happen to fall into the "other" category because of your body size, you are automatically treated differently, with your body being pathologized by the medical community. Your body is now viewed as a problem or illness which must be corrected.

It is worth noting that there is no way to adjust the BMI measurement to accommodate for the fact that women, and especially pregnant and breastfeeding women, naturally tend to have a higher amount of adipose (fat) tissue so they may nourish their developing fetus and later, feeding infant. Despite this flawed formula, BMI is still used by obstetricians, midwives and facilities worldwide to justify putting pregnant people into categories and levels of "risk."

The higher your BMI, the more likely your options for birth are to be limited and interfered with. The bigger your body, the more likely those who are meant to support you may see your birth as being a risky, dangerous endeavor. Hospitals, birth centers and even independent providers, like midwives, may have policies which limit access to services for these reasons—the most common being home birth, birth center care and access to a pool to labor and/or birth in.

Although diet culture, weight stigma and the useless body mass index have contributed to the single story of fat pregnancy, you can fight back! You can reject this narrative which pathologizes, dehumanizes and medicalizes pregnancy in a bigger body. The reality, and the story which should be told, is that people in bigger bodies can and do have positive pregnancies with healthy outcomes every single day. **You are capable of creating your own unique story.**

FAT BIRTH

Chapter Two:
FAT AND JOYFUL

In case no one has said this to you before—you are worthy of a joyful fat pregnancy! Happiness and harmony are not something reserved only for your straight size friends. You deserve to feel the excitement of growing a baby and helping that human enter the world, no matter your size and health status. You have the ability to embrace your pregnancy, your changing body and look forward to one of life's most incredible moments.

Your Pregnancy Mindset

Your mindset is essentially the collection of beliefs and attitudes you have. Think of it as a lens that helps you navigate and interpret the world around you. These attitudes and beliefs impact the decisions you make, your behavior and your internal dialogue. Your beliefs have been built upon over time, of course, but this does not mean they are unchangeable. You can get in touch with whatever belief system you have and decide whether it is beneficial for you or needs some adjusting.

When you consider your own mindset, tune into your beliefs surrounding bodies and pregnancy. Do you view pregnancy in a bigger body as inherently challenging? Do you think plus size people should be treated differently during pregnancy? What are your feelings on how one's weight may impact birth? Do you believe it is fair to create unique restrictions for people of size? Are some of your beliefs fatphobic? Are your attitudes benefiting you? How do they make you feel? Do your beliefs lean toward the *fearful fat* narrative of pregnancy, which implies fat pregnancy is more dangerous or risky? If so, what is the alternative to this mindset?

BEING UNAPOLOGETICALLY FAT AND PREGNANT!

Society may pathologize fatness, telling us it is the worst thing we can be—but buying into that bullshit is a choice. Remember, you are creating your own story and it can be one that embraces and respects your journey to becoming a parent. You do not need to apologize to yourself, your baby or anyone else for daring to be pregnant in a bigger body. You do not need to hide behind the narrow representations of pregnancy shown to us on repeat. You are allowed to take up space in a world that says fat bodies should not be seen. It is not always easy, but it is worth it.

Shifting your mindset so it is increasingly fat positive, also called size-friendly, is more of a journey than a destination. Everyone who begins moving away from one mindset to another is doing so in baby steps. If it has taken years to build and reinforce a set of beliefs, it is only realistic that change will take time—but each day is a step in a more compassionate direction. Even small steps which may seem insignificant to others can make the biggest impact for you and how you feel during pregnancy.

I hope you fall in love with your pregnant body and the amazing power it has to support the creation of life. If loving your body seems like too big of a jump right now, you can aim for body neutrality and body respect, which you will read about within these pages. If you have spent a large portion of your life trying to change your body or have felt like being fat is the worst thing in the world, changing your mindset may feel like an incredible and overwhelming shift. The ideas and concepts below are key ingredients in helping shift your mindset so you are better able to embrace your plus size pregnancy. Some of these concepts may be new to you and if so, that is completely okay! If you are familiar with these views, then I encourage you to check in with them anyway and see if you can strengthen these aspects of your mindset even further.

Fat Positive Pregnancy Mindset

- Accepting Change
- Body Neutrality
- Intuitive Eating
- Looking After Your Mental Health

ACCEPTING CHANGE

There is nothing that personifies change more than the pregnant body. It shifts, expands, grows, softens and opens as it nourishes new life. These changes happen from second to second and while many are external, what really fills me with awe are the changes happening within the body. Billions of cells multiplying, organs literally changing position to accommodate the growing womb and hormones building to a peak as birth approaches. All of this wonder, magic and intuitive connection happens within fat bodies. Your fatness does not dim or dull this experience.

Of course, during this joyous and sometimes overwhelming time, things can also be really shit. I am no stranger to the reality that pregnancy often brings a wagon-load of discomfort and misery. If you are experiencing any of the many pregnancy symptoms that make you question why being pregnant felt like a good idea in the first place, you are not alone. It is perfectly valid to be grateful to be pregnant while also admitting that you wish you could skip to the end bit when your baby is here. Some of the ways in which your body changes may be new or unsettling, especially if you have experienced any issues with body image in the past. Give yourself space to work through those feelings, rest when you need to and honor your body's needs.

SOME TYPICAL BODY CHANGES

- Blood volume increases by 40-50%
- The uterus grows to be twenty times heavier than its pre-pregnancy size at full term— 50 grams to over 1,000 grams!
- Growth of an entirely new organ: the placenta
- Varicose veins may appear as the result of the uterus compressing blood vessels
- Stretch marks may develop anywhere as the body grows and expands
- Other skin changes: the "pregnancy glow" caused by increased blood volume, acne, linea nigra on the abdomen and pigment changes on the face called melasma
- Estrogen causes maternal tissue growth in the uterus and breasts
- The hormone relaxin loosens joints and ligaments, especially those in the pelvis
- Darkening of the areolas
- Increased hormone levels: estrogen, progesterone, prolactin and human chorionic gonadotropin
- Swelling, brought on by water retention
- You start to get a pregnancy "bump"
- Changes in weight

Bodies change in whatever ways they need to during pregnancy. These changes may feel much less unsettling if viewed through the lens of non-judgment. When you observe your body, you can take note of any changes without assigning labels of "good" or "bad." Change is a part of all lived experiences and can be viewed as neutral if we choose— although this may be easier said than done. You can begin to embrace change with the knowledge that many external body changes are reflecting the magnificent shifts happening internally. Many people may struggle to accept changes their body goes through when they are *not* pregnant, so sudden changes during gestation may feel even more extreme.

Ashlee Bennett, an art therapist, counselor and author, known as The Body Image Therapist, beautifully describes how change impacts the brain:

> It's normal to feel some discomfort when your body changes, even if you've rejected diet culture and body ideals... Your brain

contains your **body image 'map'**—it's how it makes sense of your body in space and time. When your body changes, your brain receives new information about the body as you go about your life *e.g. a waist band that becomes tight...* When it receives new information, it can almost feel jarring as it's noticing a discrepancy—and this is a good thing as it's a sign your brain is updating itself with new information. The issue arises when we read into the normal discomfort of change (as the brain is updating) and start to make meaning of it and ascribe a value judgement to it, which can lead to body dissatisfaction and distress and down the spiral you go. (Original emphasis)[1]

THE ISSUE OF WEIGHT GAIN

This body change is often the most challenging for people to accept and adapt to because it is so intertwined with our own belief systems regarding body size. The Institute of Medicine (IOM) has developed weight gain recommendations for pregnancy which have been promoted by many global obstetric and health organizations. They advise that people with a BMI from 25-29.9 gain between fifteen to twenty-five pounds and for those with a BMI 30+, eleven to twenty pounds.

Medical professionals are encouraged to provide individualized care to "assist women in gaining within these guidelines"[2] and one has to wonder, what does "assist" actually mean? In many cases healthcare providers offer the oversimplified standard of "eat less, move more," while in other cases, people are fat shamed in an attempt to will them into weight loss—another tactic which does not work and has the opposite effect of causing further harm to fat folks.[3]

Weight shaming and humiliation are not and will not make people any thinner or more healthy. Pregnant people who are at the receiving end of weight stigmatizing experiences more likely to have dieting behaviors—like restricting their food intake—engage in emotional eating, feel depressed and have higher levels of stress during pregnancy.[3]

While the IOM guidelines are something to consider, ultimately, all forms of weight gain are normal and are impacted by a myriad of personal issues. Research has shown that two-thirds of pregnant mothers have been unable to stay within the arbitrary weight guidelines set by the IOM, which are also assigned solely based on the BMI metric.[4] This is evidence that Mother Nature often has her own plans that we cannot control our way out of. This has not stopped some weight-biased medical professionals from suggesting that fat folks either lose weight or "maintain" their weight during pregnancy—neither of which are recommended by the IOM. While we know actively trying to lose weight during pregnancy is not recommended, what does "maintain your weight" really mean? Lose weight. Allow me to explain.

If you consider all of the internal and external changes happening during pregnancy, you will notice many of these changes have a weight attached to them. The average person, including a plus size person, can expect to gain anywhere from twenty-five to thirty pounds as a result of these changes *which happen to every pregnant person,* regardless of their size.

- Increase in blood volume and other body fluids: 6-8 lbs
- Increase in body fat, proteins, nutrients and breast tissue: 7-9 lbs
- Uterine growth: 2 lbs
- Placenta: 1.5-3 lbs
- Amniotic fluid: 2 lbs
- The weight of your baby: 6-10 lbs

Simple math tells us if someone is, for example, 200 lbs and they maintain that weight throughout pregnancy, once their baby is born, they will be lighter as their body has time to settle postpartum. The recommendation to maintain your weight is not a neutral one, as it is only suggested to fat people through the lens of fatphobia. Furthermore, *it may encourage restriction or disordered eating* for some people who start to focus heavily on maintaining their weight at all costs. Worryingly, more than one in three expecting parents in the United States is *actively trying* to lose weight or maintain their weight during pregnancy.[5] This attempt is often made by increasing physical activity and food restriction, which may impact nutrient intake, energy levels, amniotic fluid levels (especially if dehydrated), birth weight, fetal growth and more.

This seemingly harmless recommendation, aimed at keeping fat people from getting any fatter, may have serious consequences for some. If your provider has said this to you, remember that your pregnancy does not need to revolve around your weight; some weight gain is normal for people of all sizes, you can request not to be weighed during pregnancy or have a "blind" weight taken—this is when you are weighed but the number is kept in your medical file, not to be shared with you. More importantly, the amount of weight you gain during pregnancy says *nothing* about your worth as a human being or your potential as a new parent. You are not a better person if you gain less and you are not a bad or "out of control" person if you gain more. Those fatphobic messages have no place within maternity culture, or anywhere for that matter.

Body Neutrality

If you are not in a place where you feel like you can begin loving your body, body neutrality is a wonderful way to begin reconnecting with the body you have. Body neutrality is a concept sometimes referred to as body acceptance. It is a way to engage with your body with the understanding that how you feel has nothing to do with how your body looks. It accepts that there are times when you are going to have a bad day, where you may struggle to accept different aspects of your body and this has nothing to do with your self worth. Body neutrality does not require that you even like your body. It encourages you to begin focusing on how your body functions and how your body allows you to experience life.

During pregnancy, body neutrality will help bring your attention away from how your body looks and help you rekindle an appreciation for all of the things your body *does*. It is *your body* that conceived, is sustaining your pregnancy and going through immense changes as it grows and nurtures your baby. When you engage with body neutrality, you are recognizing these changes and helping develop an appreciation for your body as it prepares for birth. Clinical nutritionist and intuitive eating expert Stephanie Dodier so brilliantly explains, "The goal of body neutrality is to dial down the enormous significance that's being given to physical beauty and attractiveness in our society... It pushes back on the complete concept that promotes beauty as essential, as consequential, as the ultimate accomplishment of a person's life."[6] When you begin your journey to body neutrality, you may find that you do not think much about your body at all, which is normal and may be a relief.

Appreciating and respecting yourself is the beginning of making peace with your body and genetics, which also impact the changes you may experience during your pregnancy. Showing your body kindness and respect includes:

- Nourishing your body with meals and snacks
- Engaging in movement that feels restorative
- Attending regular dental and medical appointments
- Self care, including rest, taking medications, hygiene, etc.
- Buying and wearing clothes that fit comfortably

INTUITIVE EATING

Intuitive eating is another way to engage with your body which will promote a relationship of kindness and self respect during pregnancy and beyond. Laura Thomas, a registered nutritionist, intuitive eating counselor and the author of *Just Eat It,* describes intuitive eating as a systemic approach to releasing food rules as well as the worry and anxiety often associated with eating.[7] Those who engage with intuitive eating re-learn how to honor their body's natural, internal cues, including: hunger, satiety, satisfaction, pleasure and peace. Intuitive eating is not something that needs to be learned as a new skill. On the contrary, *everyone was born* an intuitive eater, but somewhere along the way, many of us learned to distrust our bodies.

All babies are born knowing how to respond to hunger, when to eat and when to stop once satisfied. At some point we became fearful of our own body's signals of hunger and disconnected from feelings of fullness and satisfaction with food. Sadly, it is predicted that up to 75% of women have disregarded this innate knowledge, having turned to some form of disordered eating—often a series of diets. Diet culture promotes disordered eating, which creates chaos around food and the moral value we assign to our relationship with food.

The goal of intuitive eating is to become an "unaffected eater."[8] This entails becoming re-acquainted with how to recognize your hunger signals, learning to respect levels of fullness, allowing yourself to feel the pleasure that comes with eating food and learning to eat what you want without assigning moral value to food as "good" or "bad." When you embrace the principles of intuitive eating, you will also find that you do not feel guilt, shame or view eating as an ethical dilemma. Any preoccupation you have with food is abolished and a renewed sense of freedom emerges. If this sounds too good to be true, I am living proof that it is not. Healing from my clinical eating disorder was firmly rooted in intuitive eating.

I first discovered and welcomed intuitive eating into my life following the birth of my fourth baby, when I was thirty years old. I had spent all of my adult life doing one form or another of disordered eating. I had tried all the diets which promoted food restriction, counted calories, practiced fasting, increased my exercise and beat myself up emotionally in the process. As a fat person, I felt like it was my mission to lose weight in whatever way possible. I did not initially realize how dieting had negatively affected both my mental and physical health. My weight loss obsession was destroying my life in many ways and pulling me away from my large family and the time I spent with my children. I had become completely disconnected from my body and unable to identify feelings of hunger, fullness or satisfaction. I had become afraid to feel anything.

Intuitive eating was my journey back to myself. I spent months learning what it meant to be an intuitive eater and unlearning the absurd food rules I had created and followed over the years thanks to diet culture. I was amazed at the level of freedom I felt when I was no longer a slave to the scale, calorie counting or labeling foods as "off-limits." It was challenging to stop believing in and following all of the food rules I had tried in the past. Instead of constantly trying to change my body, I learned to accept it and nourish it with foods that fit into my life without judgment. When I paired body neutrality with intuitive eating, I began enjoying my life more, my mind was free from obsessive thoughts regarding weight loss and I became a more mindful parent.

There are so many benefits to intuitive eating and there are over twenty studies that have looked at them. The book *Intuitive Eating* has an entire chapter dedicated to summarizing the research findings, some of which include:[8]

- Higher body satisfaction
- Higher levels of body appreciation and acceptance
- More diverse diet for those who eat intuitively
- Increased levels of optimism
- Reduction in binge eating behavior
- Reduced levels of inflammation and cortisol levels in the body
- Being less likely to eat emotionally, such as in response to stress or upset

So many people have had issues with food, but we rarely talk about it. I am not here to tell you whether you do or do not have disordered eating habits, but it is worth taking note of and recognizing that if you do, *there is an alternative*. Intuitive eating will promote a deeper connection with your body and has been shown to improve overall health. Take an honest look at your own lived experiences around food and exercise. If you feel like you need more support, you may wish to seek the support of an intuitive eating counselor. Alternatively, there are entire books and self-led workbooks dedicated to intuitive eating written by experts. Please see further resources at the back of this book for titles.

WHAT DOES DISORDERED EATING LOOK LIKE?

Laura Thomas so brilliantly describes a continuum of eating, in which intuitive eating is on one end, disordered eating is in the middle and clinical eating disorders are at the opposite end of the continuum.[7] Disordered eating is the norm within the western world and it is sneakily pervasive, making it even more challenging to identify. This is evidenced by the number of common food rules, food tracking and fitness apps, magazines and books filled with dieting tips—all of which promote disordered eating and behaviors aimed at changing one's physical appearance. People who have engaged in disordered eating may currently or previously have had elaborate rules regarding when, how and what they should eat. They may have dedicated an enormous amount of time to calculating calories, counting macros and deciphering how much they need to exercise to "earn" future food or punish themselves for eating something. They may also experience a cocktail of negative emotions associated with food—guilt, shame, fear and anxiety are common. A disconnection to their body's hunger and fullness cues is the norm, along with a feeling of mistrust—"I just can't trust myself around tempting foods!"

If this sounds exhausting, it is! The constant preoccupation with food rules and looking for external validation that what you are doing is "right," can overwhelm anyone who engages in these behaviors.

Disordered eating is, of course, something that may be experienced prior to pregnancy and food rules may become heightened or reignited during pregnancy for those struggling with body-image issues. If you identify as having concerns surrounding food and physical activity, there is a way to journey back to intuitive eating in a gentle way. There are entire intuitive eating communities ready to assist you!

LOOKING AFTER YOUR MENTAL HEALTH

It is no exaggeration that pregnancy is a time filled with many new and conflicting emotions. How and when you conceive, how your pregnancy is progressing, your views on birth and expectations about new parenting may all impact your perinatal mental health. There are many avenues in which you can get support locally if needed, with many areas improving mental health services for pregnant people. If a service, such as, counseling is not available to you locally, there are many online options as well.

SET THOSE BOUNDARIES

It is important to surround yourself with people who will support you as you journey to grow your family without judgment or shame. The conversations and messages you receive from others impact how you feel and if someone is adding to your levels of stress or anxiety—or just making you feel shit about yourself for some reason—setting boundaries is key. You are the only person who gets to decide who you interact with and when. The majority of people who take issue when others set boundaries are often the most frequent boundary-crossers. When you become pregnant you may find that you have suddenly become a magnet for unsolicited advice and information, which may be laced with backhanded comments—"If I were your size, I would…"

I once attended the Self Love Summit in London where author Petra Kelly was a speaker. One of the most profound things she said, and what has stuck with me since as a chronic avoider of confrontation, was this—"Self care is setting boundaries. Self love is upholding them, no matter who it ruffles." Have truer words ever been said? So many of us set boundaries that are to our benefit, only to become slack when a few feathers are ruffled. Give yourself permission to put *you* first. Repeat this as many times as necessary. Setting boundaries does not imply you are aggressive or selfish, it means you are taking care of *you* during this special time—time you will never get back, I might add. If you have found that your closest family and friends are not the right people to support you during your pregnancy, feel free to look elsewhere. You may find better understanding in a size-friendly support group online.

GET REAL WITH YOUR SOCIAL MEDIA FEED

You do not have to go far to notice that there is a complete lack of representation of fat and pregnant bodies within our visual culture. On social media you will not see a fat pregnant body anywhere unless you are actively searching for this type of content. Fat bodies continue to be censored on many social media platforms, including Instagram, who (erroneously) cite such images violate their community standards. The hashtag #FatIsNotAViolation was created in response to Instagram removing posts and deactivating entire accounts when people shared content that featured their partially-clothed fat bodies.[9] When fat bodies *are* depicted in the media, the focus is usually on weight loss, further stigmatizing fatness. In other depictions, those featured have their heads cropped out of the images, in what has become known as "digital decapitation".[10] This editing aims to dehumanize the fat body by literally denying it a face.

What we are shown instead of pregnant bodies of all types is an unattainable "ideal"—a thin, white, cis-gendered female with a bump that is smooth, round, pronounced and devoid of any marks, including linea nigra, scars, stretch marks and common pregnancy rashes. These depictions are complete fiction because they do not exist in the real world, thanks to strategic lighting, posing, the invention of filters and editing software. It takes entire teams of people to edit, shrink, smooth, erase and change the shape of the finished products we see today. It is no wonder so many people feel their pregnancy is not something that should be celebrated, given the lack of representation and the active erasure of fat bodies.

As you look through your social media feeds, consider the type and variety of content you are consuming on a daily basis. Be honest about whether it is helpful or harmful to your body image and whether it is increasing your feelings of confidence for birth or making you feel more apprehensive. If you are following a narrow range of accounts that are highlighting the same experiences on repeat, diversifying your feed is a must. During pregnancy, I encourage my doula clients to source and follow two types of accounts: those that empower them as they prepare for birth and those that feature a range of body types. There are literally thousands that share positive information for those preparing for birth. Typical topics may include the role of informed decision-making, birth planning, tips for birth partners, birth stories, comfort measures for labor and so much more! Size-friendly accounts will show a range of body types and help normalize the joyful fat experience of birth.

CHECKING IN

With the busy-ness of life, it is common to put your own wants and needs last. I encourage you to see pregnancy as a time to prioritize yourself, which will benefit both you and your baby. These check-in questions will assist you in unearthing how you honestly feel right now.

- Am I nervous or worried about something?
- Who or what can help me through this?
- What can I do to feel prepared for my next step?
- How can I comfort myself right now?

Remember that pregnancy is a journey and taking care of yourself means making *you* a priority. While many plus size expecting parents may find they have a new level of respect and appreciation for their body, those feelings are not always automatic. The four tips below are practical ways you can begin embracing your body and your pregnancy right now.

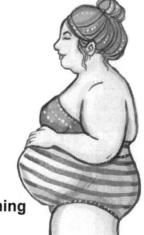

Embrace Your Pregnant Body:

- **Get in touch with your bump**
- **Document your pregnancy**
- **Get yourself comfortable clothing**
- **Joyful movement**

ONE: GET IN TOUCH WITH YOUR BUMP

So many people have felt shame about their bodies, with their bellies being a particularly criticized area. Society would have us believe that the larger your stomach, the more unhealthy you must be. Diet culture has increased soft belly hatred, with the beauty and weight loss industries constantly trying to sell and promote solutions that will sculpt and shrink this area. The "apple shape," the body type which has the fullest stomach, is often depicted as the least attractive, most stubborn and most problematic. All of this body shaming has led to a serious disconnection with our bellies.

You *can* start to embrace your belly, whether it looks like a visible "bump" or not, with baby steps. No matter your pre-pregnancy shape or size, your uterus will grow approximately forty centimeters during gestation, which will create some serious crowding of your other organs. Can we all just stop and appreciate that fact for a moment? Your other organs will literally *move* to accommodate your baby! This space that has once housed so many shameful feelings will now be your baby's loving home until birth.

Get reacquainted with this area if you have avoided looking at or touching your stomach lovingly. You can start by touching your stomach through your clothes. Imagine you are soothing your baby to sleep as you gently stroke or rub your belly in a circular motion. You may even like to sing a song or speak to your baby as you do this. By eighteen weeks, your baby will be able to hear you from inside the womb. This is a lovely way to bond with your baby and touching your bump from outside your clothing first may help you feel more comfortable with eventually touching your bare belly. Adding a special cream, oil or essential oils to the mix can create an even more special experience and promote the production of the relaxing hormone, oxytocin—which is discussed more in Chapter Six.

As your pregnancy progresses into the second trimester, you will begin to feel amazing movements made by your baby. Many plus size parents wonder if they will feel these sensations later because of their size, but that is not the case. Most first-time parents will feel their baby's first kicks by twenty-two weeks, with subsequent parents often noticing them sooner. Your weight does not impact these kicks being felt internally. You may feel less sensation, however, if your placenta is anterior—meaning it is attached to the front of your uterus. This is a normal place for the placenta to attach no matter your size, although it may mean some of your baby's movements are "cushioned" by this organ. Have no fear, as your baby continues to grow and their movements become stronger, you will definitely feel them! Many fat parents also begin to feel their baby's kicks externally in the late second or early third trimester. Feeling these kicks is another great way to connect with your baby. You can get other loved ones, such as your partner, older children, family and friends involved in feeling them if you are comfortable.

If you are looking for more of an artistic activity, you may enjoy belly casting or bump painting. Belly casting is literally a plaster cast of your pregnant belly being made with either an at-home kit or you may hire someone to help. Once completed, you can leave the cast as is or you can decorate it for display or to enjoy privately. Bump painting, either actual paint or henna, is another way you can involve others in embracing your bump. As with belly casting, you can create a memorable experience in your home or hire an artist to assist with this. Both options create a wonderful window of opportunity to get some pictures taken of your bump if you are up for it! A quick online search can help if you are stuck for ideas.

BUMP SHAPES

Many people of size wonder when they will begin showing and what their pregnancy bump will look like. When you and others begin to notice a distinctive bump depends on your shape, size, how your weight is distributed and what number pregnancy you are having. It typically takes first-time moms of all sizes longer to have a visible bump because their tissues and ligaments have not been stretched in this capacity before. Those with subsequent pregnancies often say they show weeks sooner than their first. It is also important to note that it is very common for *you to notice a difference* in your abdomen's shape and size before others will.

I noticed my own body shifting and changing very early on in my first trimester but did not begin visibly showing to others until I was well into my second. I began to feel a subtle sensation of more fullness and roundness, which other people simply could not feel or see. If you naturally have a larger waistline, it may take bit longer for you to have a visible pregnancy bump. Many people of size report that they begin showing sometime between twenty to thirty weeks.

Waiting for your bump to be more visible can be very frustrating. Many fat folks are waiting for acknowledgment from others that yes, they are pregnant! With this acknowledgment often comes more support and nurturance, even from complete strangers. Mia O'Malley, a fat positive digital creator and plus size mom, described the frustrations of her "invisible plus size pregnancy" in this way:

> You'll almost never get offered a seat on the train or some extra room to pass by in a crowded walkway. No one will think twice about bumping into you or squeezing past you. Waiters will ask you if you'd like wine with your dinner or to hear about their new cocktails... Your partner and friends may [have to] advocate on your behalf to get a seat at a crowded restaurant or bar. My friend is 7 months pregnant, can we take that seat?[11]

If you feel like your pregnancy is invisible, you are not alone. While receiving special treatment from others is a bonus, there are many ways you and your loved ones can embrace and celebrate your pregnancy no matter your bump's shape or size.

When most people envision a pregnancy bump, what they see is a D belly. From the side, this type of belly has one curve, creating the classical D shape often portrayed in the media. While this shape is typical for some, plus size parents may also have what is called a B belly, and it is perfectly normal! A B belly, sometimes called a "double belly," looks more like a B shape when you stand to the side. This bump shape often looks like there is a waistband in the middle, creating a division between the top and bottom of the belly. One's fascial health impacts the type of pregnancy bump one will develop.

Fascia is the connective tissue that forms beneath the skin and it is affected by physical activity, hydration levels, eating habits, prior injuries, previous pregnancies, stress and weight. This tissue is what ultimately influences the shape of your belly. The shape and size of your bump will also change during the course of your pregnancy so it may fluctuate between looking like a D or B, all dependent on your unique body changes. Your body is worth celebrating no matter what shape your bump is.

TWO: DOCUMENT YOUR PREGNANCY

One of the most common postpartum regrets I hear from plus size parents is that they wish they had taken more pictures of themselves during pregnancy. Many people do not capture images of their bump because they feel self-conscious about their abdomen or believe they may not "look pregnant enough." I implore you to take images documenting your pregnancy even if you feel like you do not have a visible bump or do not like how you look now. Pregnancy is a special time no matter what your body looks like and you are better off taking too many images that you can delete in the future versus having regrets that you do not have any. Your pictures may include lovely everyday shots or you can go one step further and hire a photographer to help you. No matter what type of photos you have, your child will appreciate looking back on those memories with you.

If you decide to have professional maternity pictures taken, these are some things to consider:

- **Type of Photographer:** Someone who is experienced in taking family photos, for example, is not necessarily going to rock a maternity session. Ask photographers if they have any experience photographing plus size expecting parents and ask to see their portfolio if it is not readily available online. You may also want to ask for referrals from others.
- **Gathering Your Ideas:** Look for examples of maternity photos you like. Are there colors or themes that you prefer? Do you want solo pictures, some with your partner or older children? Do you like indoor or outdoor scenes? Whatever location you decide on, consider how you will feel and if that might translate into your pictures. For example, some people may feel more anxious having photos taken outdoors where there may be onlookers, while others may not mind at all.
- **Open Communication with Your Photographer:** Discuss any concerns you may have and what poses you are most interested in. Come right out and tell your photographer if you are nervous. Maybe you have never had professional photos taken before. If you want more of an emphasis on your bump so it looks a certain way, tell them.

Maybe you want less of an emphasis on something else. These are your pictures and your maternity session, so you decide!

- **Select Your Photo Shoot Clothes:** You have envisioned your maternity wear, now it is time to find it! This is completely individual. Some people prefer dresses of different styles from flowy to form fitting, lingerie emphasizing their bare bump or swimwear, and others may be fully nude. Do and wear whatever makes you feel the most comfortable and feels the most like you.
- **Be Organized:** Having your location and outfit already decided means you will be able to envision your photo session in advance. You will also be less stressed on the day so you can get ready feeling more calm and confident.
- **Don't Forget to Have Fun!** You will of course remember to smile but do not be afraid to laugh during your photo session, too. Take breaks when you need to, bring some water to stay hydrated and remember to just be you. You do not need to pretend to be a model or do unnatural poses for the camera. Oftentimes the best pictures are snapping those organic movements and facial expressions.

THREE: GET YOURSELF SOME COMFORTABLE CLOTHING

Finding clothes that are available, affordable and appealing to you can be incredibly challenging if you are plus size and pregnant. All people of size know the range of standard clothing is already limited and sadly, it is even more so when it comes to maternity clothes. The range of what is available often depends on your location and of course, your budget. It is typical for many maternity brands carrying larger sizes to either only be online, or for those who are brick and mortar, their plus size maternity ranges may be solely online. If you are someone who likes to try on clothing or are working with a budget, this is incredibly frustrating. No one should have to deal with spending more money on shipping, returns, customs charges and the other costs associated with being forced to purchase everything online. If you are someone who is super plus size, many brands may not carry your size. All I can say about this is it is *incredibly unfair and I am sorry.* All fat people deserve cute clothing that makes them feel comfortable while looking great. I wish I could tackle this problem, but all I can offer are some suggestions.

Firstly, search high and low. Look for shops in your area and even look in secondhand shops. Maternity clothes are only worn for a short time so they may not have had much wear and you can snag yourself a bargain. If your favorite store does have maternity clothes but they are all online, see if you can order directly to the store and avoid any additional shipping or return fees if desired. Secondly, go crazy on the internet. Check the shops you usually peruse but do not be afraid to branch out and try others you may not have heard of and even for-sale groups on social media. There are loads of parents of size who empathize with the true struggle of finding maternity clothes in larger sizes. They will often sell on large stashes of clothes to other parents who are having difficulty sourcing some in their area.

If you do not have any luck finding clothing that is not going to break the bank, it is perfectly okay to try to size up in the brands you already wear. This is easier to do with clothing that is already open or flowy— dresses, larger tank tops, cardigans and more. This is obviously not ideal in some circumstances and some clothing can prove to be too baggy in the chest if you size up to accommodate your abdomen, but I encourage you to get creative and ultimately choose whatever makes you feel great. You can also wear your pre-pregnancy clothes longer with an adjustment or two. Some people go complete DIY sewing diva on their pants and other bottoms to add panels that stretch. Others buy a stretchy band, sometimes called a belly band, that will slip over unzipped pants, allowing them to be worn unzipped without showing any skin. This can add weeks or even months of life to your clothing. When all else fails, get yourself an incredible pair of stretchy maternity leggings and wear them every damn day until the inner thighs are worn.

FOUR: JOYFUL MOVEMENT

Joyful movement is intuitive movement. It is listening to your body during pregnancy and honoring both your body's need to rest and engage in physical activity when you need and want to. There are many myths associated with activity and I encourage you to release them all. For starters, you do not need to torture yourself to reap the benefits of movement. Physical activity is meant to rejuvenate the body, not deplete it. Driving yourself into the ground can potentially cause injury, especially with that relaxin hormone coursing through your body. Always consider your limits, your hydration level and how any activity is making you feel both physically and emotionally. Only you know when you are doing too much or have reached a limit. Stop when you need to, even if that means doing less activity than you may have last week, last month or before you conceived. This is another area where expecting parents can sometimes start comparing themselves to prior activity levels or what other people are doing. This is your body and your pregnancy, not anyone else's. As with your changing body, try not to associate the feelings of "good" or "bad" with your movement. Whatever you are doing is enough if it feels right for you.

Physical activity is often associated with weight loss goals and tracking, tracking, tracking. Neither of these things need to be a priority for you and I implore you to disconnect movement, weight and food altogether. You will notice that I am not using the word "exercise," because I often feel like it is so closely tied to weight loss and diet culture—both of which promote counting of all sorts. You may be familiar with the length of time you were active, the number of calories burned and the distance you cycled, walked or ran. When you detach yourself from these numbers and start to focus on how you *feel*, movement can be so much more enjoyable.

BENEFITS

When you shift your focus away from exercise-associated numbers, it is much easier to hone in on what movements feel right for you and exactly *how* they make you feel. Are you feeling more energized? Have your stress levels gone down? Does movement give you space and time to think so you feel more clear-headed? Has your sleep improved? These are just some of the benefits you may experience. Movement may also be particularly helpful to ease common aches and pains experienced during pregnancy, including back pain, round ligament pain and constipation. Many of these common ailments can be eased with gentle movement, such as stretches, prenatal yoga, water aerobics or other techniques recommended by a physiotherapist specializing in maternity support.

Physical activity has other benefits for both expecting parents and babies. During pregnancy, moderate activity lowers the likelihood of developing maternal high blood pressure and preeclampsia.[12] Another study showed that there is a 34% reduction of gestational diabetes when expecting parents take brisk walks three to four times a week.[13] Psychological benefits include reduced feelings of depression, anxiety and a reduction in the production of the stress hormone, cortisol.[14] For those who have been diagnosed with gestational diabetes, research has shown that moderate to high levels of physical activity can assist with treatment and reduce the need for insulin use.[15]

The benefits of physical activity continue to carry over into the birth space with reductions seen in rates of instrumental deliveries, via forceps or vacuum-assisted, and cesarean birth by sixteen percent.[16] This reduction in cesarean rates was found when expecting parents engaged in aerobic movement lasting thirty to sixty minutes and occurring between two and seven times per week.[12] For those who continued regular physical activity into the third trimester, they were more likely to have a shorter labor.[17]

MAKE ACTIVITY FUN

- Choose an activity you enjoy
- Explore other activities you may not have done prior to pregnancy
- Listen to music, audiobooks or hypnobirthing tracks during movement
- Link up with a friend or family member to make activity a more social experience or, alternatively, go solo if you need time and space to yourself
- Don't forget to wear comfortable clothing!
- Join a size-friendly class either online or in-person

If going to the gym is not your style, engaging in activities outdoors or online from home is another great option. You may seek pregnancy-specific classes, such as yoga or pilates, while other standard classes are often appropriate too with some minor adjustments. There has been an increasing number of fat fitness instructors on social media who share a plethora of free and low-cost content. MissFits Workout® offers online and in-person "dance inspired group exercise classes for those who don't feel at home in the gym" and founder Becky has incredible, inspiring fat positive content online as well.[18] Most physical activity is fine to engage in during pregnancy, so long as you avoid those which may lead to collisions or falling. Water aerobics is one of my personal favorites, as it is an excellent way to release muscle tension, stretch the body and the buoyancy is a wonderful relief from the added heaviness that pregnancy can bring to bodies of any size. If you are unsure about when and what types of movement are ideal for you, always get in touch with your healthcare provider for more clarification.

Truly wonderful things can happen when you reevaluate your mindset and begin embracing your plus size pregnancy without judgment. You will begin to accept and appreciate your body more. It will become easier to honor your body's needs and recognize your limits. You will notice that your confidence begins to grow as you approach birth. Any fears or worries you may have had can be completely eliminated or reduced significantly. No matter where you are in your journey toward a more fat positive pregnancy and birth, I hope you remember that even small steps make a big impact.

Within this text, you will find affirmations, like the one below, which will serve as reminders of the incredible things your body is doing right now. You can also head over to www.fatandpregnant.com/shop and enter code **FATBIRTHBOOK** to get your free body positive affirmations MP3 that you can listen to throughout pregnancy whenever you need an extra boost.

Each day I nurture myself so I may nurture my baby

Chapter Three:
BOSS YOUR BIRTH

Something I have observed with frustration during my time as a doula and childbirth educator is how commonplace it is for expecting parents to hand over the reins of their experience to another person—oftentimes a medical professional. In all other settings where we want to or need to access medical care, we accept and understand our right to bodily autonomy. For some reason when it is time to birth our babies, we hand over full responsibility and control to someone else. Experts in birth, whether they be doctors, midwives, obstetric nurses, doulas or other birth professionals can be a great source of comfort, wisdom and information. However, *you* are the only person who has the right to make informed decisions about what happens to your body and your baby. The decisions *you* make will have the biggest impact on your birth experience and how you enter life as a new parent.

What currently happens all too often is a birthing person will give "consent" for an examination, procedure or intervention without being truly informed. A health provider makes a recommendation, gives one reason to justify it and the expecting parent agrees without question. In doing so, the birthing person is unaware of any potential risks and the path their labor may now take. One intervention leads to another—*called the cascade of interventions*—and the new mother leaves her experience feeling stressed, violated and at its worst, traumatized. "I did not realize that agreeing to X could lead to Y."

Many new parents find themselves trying to understand exactly what happened during their birth, why things felt out of control and how they became so distanced from the decision-making process. Many return home with no explanations, assuming the care they received was inevitable and there was nothing they could have done to change the outcome.

This is a complex issue, but I believe there are three main reasons why we assume a role of passivity once we enter the birth space:

- **Culture of Compliance:** We are socialized from a young age to respect authority, do what we are told and "behave." Confrontation is often discouraged while compliance and being passive are portrayed as more favorable attributes—especially for young girls and women. As we get older, this extends to those in white coats. We "follow doctor's orders," assume "doctor knows best" and we are told not to raise any grievances even when things go wrong.
- **Hierarchy of Birth:** Expecting parents often believe that their needs and feelings are insignificant and at the very bottom of what is referred to as the "hierarchy of birth." They view healthcare professionals as experts and thus, may not feel qualified to challenge a medical recommendation or even ask questions about their own care. The reality is expecting parents are at the top of this hierarchy because they are the service-users. It is their body and their baby who are seeking care, so their needs are of the utmost importance.
- **Permission-Seeking Language:** This phenomenon illustrates the imbalance of power within the birth space. It includes both language of "allowance," permission-granting and when interventions are done under the guise of implied consent, such as:

"They told me I could not have skin to skin since I was having a cesarean."

"Because I wanted a VBAC (vaginal birth after cesarean), they told me I had to get an early epidural 'just in case.'"

"I was not allowed to have a water birth because of my BMI."

"They would not let me go past my due date, so they booked me in for induction."

"Hop up on the bed there and we'll see how dilated you are."

"I am just making a little cut," as an episiotomy is performed.

"Now we'll break your waters and move things along."

Being the boss of your body and your birth is a fundamental aspect of pregnancy and labor. It is often assumed that this human right is given within the birth space, however, there are countless stories detailing how expecting parents have been met with resistance when they began to assert themselves. This is most commonly experienced when the decisions being made are going against a common protocol, procedure or guideline. We desperately need to shift the focus of decision-making. Owning your experience does not automatically mean that there has to be an atmosphere of confrontation. You can contribute to an atmosphere of mutual respect—where you respect the feedback and recommendations you receive and your medical providers, in turn, respect your right to bodily autonomy and your ability to decide what feels right for you. Providers do not need to agree with you, but they absolutely should be providing you with respectful care no matter what you decide.

My body is growing and supporting my baby perfectly

You have the ability to ask questions and seek clarification whenever an examination, treatment or intervention is offered. You can insist (not request) that you always be involved in your care and that you be consulted before anything is done to your body. This is not to say, nor am I suggesting, that you decline everything offered to you. On the contrary, you may decide to agree with every recommended course of action, and that is okay! At least you know you have reached that decision having had the time and space to consider what feels right for you at that moment. Making your own decisions, even if they are hard ones, can add to feelings of empowerment and feeling more in control, even during difficult circumstances.

Part of owning your pregnancy is accepting that some form of preparation is required. We spend many hours preparing for life's other significant events, including weddings, holidays, important exams and more. For some reason people assume very little preparation is needed for the actual birth part—they believe everything will fall into place once labor begins. You would never turn up to your driving test without having taken a driving lesson or knowing the rules of the road—and the same holds true for birth. Knowledge is power and you are much more likely to have a positive birth experience if you have learned about the process, the current state of maternity care, what you can expect as a person of size and how you can make decisions that will improve your experience significantly. In Chapter Five you will learn more about self advocacy, the foundations of informed decision-making and how to create a birth plan that works for you.

THE OVER-MEDICALIZATION OF (FAT) BIRTH

Many expecting parents create a birth plan to help indicate what wishes they want carried out during labor, however, this document may also be reflective of what birthing people do *not* want—usually unnecessary interventions, which have become more common during birth. When you know what the reality of maternity care looks like today, you can better decide what you want to opt into and what you want to decline.

There are many people who would argue that there is no reason to try to limit interventions because they are only recommended when truly necessary anyway. This belief opposes the mountain of research which shows the exact opposite. The level of unnecessary interventions has only increased along with the introduction of more technological equipment, creating a culture of "high tech birthing".[1]

The over-medicalization of maternity care has a complicated past that has expanded globally and developed over centuries. This dramatic shift in the way people approach birth cannot be attributed to a single act or one individual. To analyze how birth has become so overly reliant on technology, we must first peer through a window into the past. This brief history is of course not all-inclusive and focuses mainly on the changes in maternity culture based in the United States and western Europe.

The medicalized model of maternity care which is the norm today has ultimately been driven by two very powerful things: patriarchy and profits.

Prior to the sixteenth and seventeenth centuries, birth was female-led and attended by "midwives" who were often local women who had given birth themselves, had witnessed births and were educated to be able to assist others. They were often viewed as "medicine women" historically with a wide array of knowledge, often including herbalism. Birth was viewed as both a social and emotional event that occurred within the home with the support of family and friends.[2] Before the invention of forceps in seventeenth-century England, men were only involved in the most difficult births.

In the early 1600s, forceps were first invented by Peter Chamberlen, who was a well-known "barber surgeon." Barber surgeons were men considered the experts of both grooming and medical procedures which standard physicians refused to do in Europe during the Middle Ages and into the Renaissance. Their knack of handling sharp instruments made them the most-suited performers of bloodletting, amputation, tooth extraction, the lancing of infections, other invasive surgeries and yes, assisting at births with obstructed babies who would not descend. With the invention of forceps, an obstructed baby was more likely to be delivered alive, so long as the parents could afford to pay the barber surgeon the hefty price—the equivalent of five thousand British pounds today.

Despite forceps being a measure which could have saved the countless lives of mothers and babies, it was a closely guarded secret by the Chamberlen family for more than two centuries. If a mother was having difficulties during labor, the forceps would be brought to the private home via a carriage. Two men would bring a large wooden box into the home, giving the illusion that forceps were a large, complicated piece of equipment. The laboring woman would then be left alone with the two men and blindfolded to help protect the family invention.[3]

By the 1880s the forceps secret was out, physicians had developed similar types and they were now being used in the western world. Male doctors quickly realized that they could make incredible amounts of money if forceps became routinely used during birth—and this is exactly what happened. Obstetricians began using them without medical need and sometimes before women were fully dilated to ten centimeters. These women were given extensive episiotomies and their babies were pulled from their bodies.

The use of forceps has had lasting effects within maternity culture, having contributed to the normalization of episiotomies and the lithotomy position, giving birth on one's back. While this position was convenient for forceps use and is still preferred by many healthcare providers today, it adds to the difficulty of the birthing person by narrowing their pelvic outlet and forcing them to literally push their baby "uphill" and against gravity. While forceps certainly did have the ability to save lives, especially for women who suffered from physical complications like rickets, they also had the potential to cause serious harm to both mothers and their babies when overused. By the 1920s forceps were routinely used and recommended for uncomplicated births in the United States.[4] Sadly this was not the last time profits would be prioritized over fetal and maternal health.

Men entering the birth world in the United States in the early 1900s can be viewed as nothing less than a patriarchal takeover with both power and profits at the helm. The tragic story of male obstetricians moving to dominate the birth market, and fill their pockets, involved taking out their midwife competitors and crushing the tradition of midwifery. Until as late as the, mid-1930s most births in the United States were attended by a midwife and happened within the home. Midwifery had become a formal profession, with knowledge continuing to be passed down with formal education programs and apprenticeships.[4] European midwives brought the knowledge they gained over generations to the USA through immigration, while Black "granny" or "grand" midwives used their birth knowledge to support pregnant people in the Old South. Indigenous midwives also attended births within their own communities before white men stepped in to both control and profit from birth.

Male obstetricians would use both sexism and racism as the base of their strategic national propaganda campaign to discredit midwives in the United States, depicting them as foreign, uneducated, dirty and an inferior choice. All of this misinformation was being disseminated at a time when midwives were providing safer care with fewer maternal deaths than doctors. These predominantly white physicians had enormous social, political and financial power behind them to further their demolition mission. Soon, wealthy females were birthing in hospitals, unaware that they were actually more likely to suffer harm due to higher rates of intervention. Another blow to midwifery was the systematic changes to both state laws and restrictions which eventually made it exceedingly challenging, if not illegal, for midwives to attend births. Within thirty years, the majority of births had moved from homes to hospitals, with male obstetricians having created a profitable, if unethical, birth monopoly for themselves.

With the majority of births in the United States now taking place in hospital settings by the early-mid 1900s, birth became pathologized and evolved into a medical event. "Care was provided as if the maternity process was a pathological dysfunction rather than biologically healthy and normal."[2] As doctors became the prominent figures within the labor room, technology began entering the birth space more heavily, as witnessed with the invention of forceps, twilight sleep and general anesthesia. Other important medical developments were also taking place during the nineteenth and twentieth centuries, including cesarean surgery and safe blood transfusions,[2] which also continued to push midwives out of the birth market. "While the shift was of enormous benefit to high-risk mothers and babies, it subjected low-risk mothers to a battery of interventions that are often counterproductive to healthy labor and delivery."[4]

While there was an initial reduction in pregnancy complications and deaths over time, especially for those mothers who were high-risk, these cannot solely be attributed to the increased use of interventions within hospital settings. The reduction in maternal mortality can also be attributed to improved overall health. Pregnant individuals had gained access to better nutrition and saw an increase in their standard of living. There were also improvements in disease control, including the importance of hand washing to reduce rates of puerperal fever in 1847.[1]

TWILIGHT SLEEP

Twilight sleep was a combination of morphine and the amnesiac scopolamine which was given to women during labor. It allowed them to remain in a state of consciousness during birth, but they were left with no memory of it. This practice was used in Europe and was popular in the United States from approximately 1914 to 1970s. The development and roll out of twilight sleep began during the same time as many suffrage movements, with women also seeking more agency over their bodies. Twilight sleep could only be given in hospital settings and thus, this demand would contribute to a further step away from the midwifery model of care.

While women who underwent twilight sleep remembered nothing, their birth was anything but a tranquil experience. Birthing people were kept in a padded crib-type bed, were blindfolded, had cotton wool placed in their ears and were restrained. Their births were distressing, often characterized by screaming that went on for hours, which they simply had no memory of. New parents started experiencing more birth injuries, they began having horrible flashbacks and suffered increased rates of maternal death as a result of twilight sleep. The medication given also impacted newborns who were more likely to need resuscitation and were often unable to effectively breastfeed. This was a result of their own sedation from the drugs used in twilight sleep that crossed the placenta. The trend declined in popularity when these side effects for moms and babies began to emerge. When twilight sleep began to be phased out, the epidural became its replacement in the 1960s.[4]

Although the twilight sleep era is behind us, its ramifications are still being felt today. Twilight sleep perpetuated the belief that birth is both a mechanical process and one that does not require consent. It gave absolute control to obstetricians who no longer saw a need to seek consent for *anything* that happened in the labor room.

Twilight sleep also reduced women to pregnant vessels which simply needed to be rid of a baby, however that might take place. Just as with the routine use of forceps, women undergoing twilight sleep were expected to lie in bed during their labor with their legs in stirrups—which could be viewed as another modern form of restraint. During twilight sleep, overly sedated women had a significantly high-risk of vomiting and aspirating the contents of their stomach, leading to death. To counteract this, physicians simply refused any nourishment. The practice of limiting food for laboring people is still common in many hospitals today, despite advancements in sedation which have improved safety.

Further developments in obstetric practice promoted increases in intervention rates, including the Friedman's Curve and active management of labor. Friedman's Curve was developed by Dr Emanuel Friedman in 1955 when he studied how long it took women to dilate and the overall length of their labors. He then plotted these points on a graph and physicians all over the world began using the Friedman's Curve to define what a "normal" labor looks like. This became problematic because there are many factors that can lengthen or shorten the labor process. If an expecting parent in a hospital setting was not laboring in the same narrow pattern defined by Dr Friedman, they were often diagnosed with "failing to progress." This diagnosis could then be used to justify the augmentation of labor by releasing someone's waters or through the use of synthetic oxytocin (Pitocin or syntocinon). Although many organizations discourage the use of this outdated form of measure today, there are many professionals who continue to rely upon it, leading to further interventions and increased cesarean rates.

Active management of labor was developed in the 1960s by Professor

Kieran O'Driscoll at the National Maternity Hospital in Dublin, Ireland. This system of literal labor management has been the subject of controversy and debate since it initially reverberated across the globe following its creation. While the acknowledged aim of active management of labor is to prevent prolonged labor for first-time moms, it also addresses the issues of cost, time and staffing allocation within busy hospital settings.[5]

The principal points of active management include:

- The diagnosis of a precise "beginning" of labor.
- The guarantee of labor not lasting longer than twelve hours. If a birthing person is not dilating at the rate of 1 cm per hour after their cervix has reached 3 cm dilated, routine amniotomy (releasing of the waters) is performed.
- If dilation is still not at the rate of 1 cm per hour, synthetic oxytocin will be administered.
- The progress of labor is charted on a graph, called a partogram.
- Once the expecting parent has entered established labor, they will receive continuous care from a midwife or other medical professional.

Active management is criticized due to its interventionist approach to all uncomplicated pregnancies, some calling it an attempt to rigidly control the birth process. It is also problematic in that it assumes a shorter labor is beneficial and safer for both moms and babies. It actively reduces birthing people down to plotted points on a graph, with all first-time moms expected to conform to a strict schedule of cervical dilation.

Research has shown women dilate at varying rates and often slower than 1 cm per hour.[6] As a result, the interventions used to expedite labor to try and meet this target are inappropriate. The "1 cm per hour ideal" set by active management of labor further pathologizes birth, creating categories of "normal" and "abnormal," leaving no room for the common biorhythms of birthing people who may wish to rest, eat or recuperate in other desired ways during labor. It is also well known that both the releasing of a mother's waters and synthetic oxytocin often increase the intensity of labor, which may lead to further interventions in the form of pain relief.

Friedman's Curve and active management of labor have had lasting implications on the way maternity care is provided today. Western culture, which values efficiency and productivity, openly supports systems put in place to increase the speed of labor. This can be problematic especially for plus size expecting parents, as some research indicates that the early stages of labor may be slower for those with a higher BMI.[7] A potentially slow first stage of labor is not "abnormal" or problematic in and of itself, although it may be referenced when recommendations for intervention are made. This notable trend, of routinely trying to speed up the labor process, is referred to as a medical provider's "failure to wait" for labor to progress on its own.

I think it is important to acknowledge that these attempts by men to both control and profit from birth have brought some significant medical advancements which have been life-saving for moms and babies. Interventions within the birth space are not negative in and of themselves. There are times when they are truly necessary to support a birthing person and their baby, as birth will never be straight forward for everyone. There should be no shame or guilt attached to wanting or requiring assistance during labor that is beneficial or may even be life-saving. Interventions become problematic, however, when they are unwanted or unnecessary to begin with and cascade into further interventions which compromise the health of mother and child. Such treatments were designed to help families, not cause more harm by their routine use.

BIRTH TODAY

Birth today continues to be characterized by high rates of intervention, with the highest levels seen within hospital settings. Statistical trends have shown a steady increase in most forms of intervention, including: amniotomy (artificial releasing of waters), electronic fetal monitoring, forceps use, vacuum-assisted delivery and cesarean birth.[2] Routine interventions during labor that were once selected for use only when needed have now been applied to all women and have become the norm. It has become increasingly rare to hear of anyone giving birth without some form of intervention.

From 2006 to 2017 the cesarean rate in the United States rose by fifty-three percent.[8] An increase in cesarean rates has also been seen globally, with more than fifteen countries having surgical birth rates higher than forty percent.[9] Rates in labor induction have also increased in many countries, including the UK where hospitals have reported 31% of mothers have their labors medically induced.[10] One study in the United States indicated the following intervention rates:[11]

- 41% of mothers had their labor begin through medical induction
- 83% used one or more forms of medication for pain relief
- Epidurals and spinal analgesia were the most common forms of pain relief, being used by 67% of people
- 31% of mothers had a cesarean birth

As routine intervention rates have increased during labor, such as the use of continuous electronic fetal monitoring, synthetic oxytocin use and routine IV fluid administration, so too have births ending with the use of forceps, ventouse and cesarean surgery. Increased risks of cesarean birth have been seen especially with moms who are induced with a low Bishop Score,[12] which is used to assess the "favorability" of the cervix. People of size also experience higher rates of cesarean birth. Research has indicated this may be due in part to provider attitudes and anti-fat bias. For example, healthcare providers suggest moving to a cesarean birth much sooner during labor when the person is plus size.[13] This means fat folks are given less time to see if labor will progress on its own, or with the use of augmentation techniques, before moving to a cesarean birth.

An increased reliance on testing, monitoring and technology is also apparent within the realm of fat pregnancy. People of size frequently share that their experiences feel even more high tech and medicalized. They may be encouraged to undergo additional glucose tolerance tests for gestational diabetes, have a higher number of ultrasounds in the third trimester and receive additional non-stress tests based on their BMI alone. One has to wonder why the end of fat pregnancies, which are often classed as "low-risk," are still being monitored so intensely.

Continuous electronic fetal monitoring (CEFM), was first introduced to delivery rooms in the 1970s, despite it not being proven to increase healthy outcomes for moms or babies at the time. It quickly moved to being another intervention that is now commonly used with all birthing people in hospital settings, although obstetric researchers believe it should be reserved only for pregnancies that are categorized as "high-risk".[2] CEFM is the most common form of fetal monitoring used in the United States today although research outcomes do not support this technology being used during low-risk pregnancies.[14,15] The overuse of this monitoring, which is done continuously while two straps are around the maternal abdomen, has consequences for both birthing people and their babies.

Firstly, it requires expecting parents to be immobile in order to collect an accurate reading and it has a high rate of false positives.[16] Thankfully, many studies have been done regarding this technology since the 1970s, which have shown CEFM is associated with a significant increase in maternal infection, instrumental vaginal birth and cesarean surgery.[16] These increased risks are seen across birthing people of all body types, including fat folks. With all of these increased risks for moms, one would assume this type of continuous monitoring would at least be beneficial for babies, however, that would be an inaccurate assumption. The use of CEFM has not reduced rates of cerebral palsy or infant mortality and research has shown it is not a good measure of neonatal wellbeing.[16] This technology has been proven to be ineffective at both identifying and predicting neurological complications in infants. Its routine use makes it one of the most debated interventions in the birth world, with some researchers calling the technology "junk science" and "rubbish technology." [17, 18] So why is continuous electronic fetal monitoring routinely used if it does not improve outcomes for moms and babies? We revert back to litigation fears and healthcare providers viewing the CEFM printed trace as protection in the event a birth-injury case arises.[19]

One alternative continuous electronic fetal monitoring is intermittent auscultation, which requires the use of a Pinard fetal stethoscope or handheld doppler to assess fetal health at timed intervals during labor. This form of monitoring allows for freedom of movement, is easy and is not associated with the increased risks that continuous electronic fetal monitoring is. The difference in cesarean rates is quite staggering when CEFM and intermittent auscultation were compared. In a 2016 study, expecting parents who had continuous electronic fetal monitoring were 63% more likely to have a cesarean those who received only intermittent auscultation. [20]

Intermittent auscultation is a safe and acceptable form of fetal monitoring which can be used during plus size birth and if this is your preference, you should definitely include it in your birth plan. This form of fetal monitoring is the standard in birth centers and at home births for pregnant people of all sizes.

TOO MUCH, TOO SOON

One of the world's most prestigious medical journals, *The Lancet,* has drawn attention to the "too much too soon" (TMTS) approach to labor, which "describes the routine over-medicalisation of normal pregnancy and birth. TMTS includes unnecessary use of non-evidence-based interventions, as well as the use of interventions that can be life saving when used appropriately, but harmful when applied routinely or overused."[21] While TMTS is typically ascribed to high-income countries, this approach is also seen in both low and middle-income areas. It leads to the increased potential harm of mothers and babies and increases healthcare costs as one intervention tends to lead to another.[21]

"Too much too soon" also describes the type of "defensive medicine" healthcare providers are encouraged to practice to avoid potential litigation. The two interventions used most by doctors to address possible litigation concerns are induction and cesarean surgery, as both give providers a larger sense of control.[1] Provider attitudes play into the increasingly high rates of cesarean births seen today, as does the overall culture of individual hospital labor wards. How a ward uses technology, the attitudes and beliefs of staff, managers' "risk tolerance" and even the design of the ward itself all impact how decisions are made and when a cesarean may be recommended.[22]

Obstetrician and researcher Neel Shah, who has studied the many reasons cesarean rates vary so much between hospitals, states, "The biggest factor in whether a woman will have a caesarean delivery 'is the door she walks through' to give birth."[22] A good way to assess the overall attitude towards birth at a specific facility or with an individual provider is to take a look at their birth statistics. What is their rate of induction, instrumental delivery and cesareans? You can compare this to other facilities, midwifery practices and providers in your area to help you decide where and how you want to access maternity care. If you are hoping for a low-intervention experience, for example, you may decide you don't want to labor at a facility whose cesarean rate is double neighboring hospitals.

I think it is important to emphasize that we have inherited a maternity situation that has historically been challenging for expecting parents and their families. This reality can feel very bleak and disempowering, however, it is important to understand the challenges within maternity culture today so you can be prepared for them, should they arise. While intervention rates continue to increase and weight stigma may, unfortunately, influence aspects of your care, do not let these facts deter you in preparing for the type of birth *you* want. Knowledge is power and there are many ways you can prepare for the positive, joyful birth that you want and deserve. The next chapter is filled with practical tips for navigating maternity care.

Chapter Four:
PREPARING FOR YOUR POSITIVE BIRTH

There are many studies which have looked at what parents want from their experiences of pregnancy and birth. Research in this area is essential so expecting parents can be supported adequately and so more focus can be brought to the improvement of maternity services. The only way to know what expecting parents want and what helps foster a positive birth is *to ask them.*

The wish for a positive pregnancy and birth is felt by pregnant people all over the world. It extends across all continents, cultures and socioeconomic contexts.[1] In short, birth matters! When thirty-five studies were analyzed from nineteen different countries, researchers found that what mattered *most* to women was a positive birth experience, which they hoped would exceed their expectations.[2] This included giving birth to a healthy baby within an environment where they felt safe. The mothers also wanted practical and emotional support, respect, reassurance and competence of their birth team.[2] While the expecting parents understood that birth is unpredictable and they may need to avail of interventions they had not anticipated, they also wanted to maintain some control through active decision-making with their care providers. Birthing people also wanted access to information in a timely manner, as it related to their individual situation.[1]

I am prepared for whatever birth my body and my baby need

A positive birth is not defined by what is written on paper. It is so much more than a description of events within a medical file. A positive birth is determined on an individual level and is based on how a person *feels* following labor and birth. It also extends beyond the physical body and its recovery. While this certainly impacts how people feel regarding their birth, it is important to understand that it is not, by any stretch of the imagination, the full picture.

Sometimes it is helpful to explore what a positive birth is *not*. A positive birth is not a prescribed sequence of events or a certain "type" of birth. A low-intervention birth and one requiring more medical intervention can *both* be viewed as positive. Two people may also have gone through similar experiences, with the same types of interventions and walk away from their births feeling completely different about it. What we miss by only considering someone's medical file is *how they were made to feel* during birth. Were they treated with dignity and respect? Did they feel involved in their care? Were they given all the information needed to make choices freely? How were any elements of fear or anxiety addressed on the day? If we only look at the physical aspects of birth, we erroneously ignore the emotional side—which is just as important.

All That Matters Is A Healthy Baby

This well-meaning phrase has to be one of the most harmful and dismissive within the birth and postpartum world. Now seen as somewhat cliché, this phrase is often said to either shut down or attempt to smooth over a birth experience that was challenging or even traumatic. It goes without question that, yes, the birth of a healthy baby is the most important thing. HOWEVER, that is not all that matters. These two beliefs, that the health of the baby is the priority, and that other aspects of the birth are important too, can exist simultaneously. Reducing birth to, "At least you have a healthy baby," or the equally problematic, "You will forget all about the birth once your baby is in your arms," is wrong and damaging.

Birthing people matter too! By implying that a healthy baby is all that matters, the voices of new parents and how they are treated during birth are silenced. Their feelings are diminished to being unimportant and even trivial. If someone needs or wants to express their dissatisfaction with their birth, they very often receive the message that they have no right to do so—*they have a healthy baby, after all. So what's the big deal?*

When the baseline of maternity services is survival, also called "health," we need to consider what that actually means. Is a "healthy baby" simply an alive one? What about the mother? By prematurely labeling all parents and babies with a pulse "healthy," society completely ignores the complex relationship being fostered between them during the earliest postpartum days and weeks, often called the fourth trimester. If a person leaves birth feeling physically and emotionally broken, we must consider how this will affect their baby. "At least you have a healthy baby," leaves no room for those considerations or discussions.

People *do care* about how they are treated and what happens to them during birth, but they may struggle to express this within a culture that pushes the belief that anything that happens in the delivery room is acceptable—so long as no one dies. If an expecting parent does suggest that they want more than a living baby, they are quickly brought down a peg, as they are accused of wanting too much or putting their "experience" ahead of their unborn child's wellbeing. Let's be clear: Parents are not being selfish or delusional if they are seeking a positive birth *and* a healthy baby. *Both* are possible and it is time we started aiming higher than survival within maternity care.

How a woman is spoken to and treated during labor is more important than the mode of delivery. This is why someone who plans a low-intervention hospital birth can still walk away feeling strong and empowered, even if more interventions or a cesarean become necessary. When people are treated with dignity, respect and are involved in their own care, those challenging times may be easier to get through and reflect upon later.

POSITIVE BIRTH, FAT BIRTH STYLE:

- Birthing in a safe environment
- Feeling supported physically and emotionally during birth
- Receiving respectful, dignified care, free of weight stigma
- Maintaining a sense of control through informed decision-making
- Access to evidence-based information

Your Team

Two of the biggest decisions you will make during your pregnancy are where you choose to give birth and who will be supporting you on the day. These decisions are often some of the first ones made, as most parents are eager to start their prenatal care within the first trimester. Knowing your options is critical, as well as knowing the advantages of choosing one over the other. The types of care available to you often depends on your location, and of course, insurance and financial constraints may play into the equation. Different forms of care will suit some and not others, so it is important to consider where and what type of provider will best support the type of experience you are trying to create.

MODELS OF CARE

There are two main models of care that exist within maternity culture, and they differ significantly. The first is the medical model, which is the dominant form in the United States. Within this model, doctors manage the care of expecting families who will most often give birth within a hospital. Physicians are encouraged to follow the general protocols and policies that have been established by the hospital in which they operate. There is often a heavier focus on preventing, diagnosing and treating any complications which may arise during pregnancy or birth. While each individual provider has their own beliefs and philosophies regarding birth, a higher reliance on testing and interventions is typical. Within this model of care, doctors are much more likely to view and treat labor as something which needs to be managed.

Obstetric-led care may be the ideal option for you for a variety of reasons. Your health history or any current health concerns may warrant birth within a hospital under specialist care. Having a higher BMI does not automatically class you as "high-risk" or mean obstetric-led care is your only option. For some people, being under the care of an obstetrician and birthing in a hospital is what makes them feel the safest. This is not "right" or "wrong," it is an understandable personal preference.

Others may opt for obstetric-led care because it is the only option for care in their area or obstetricians are the only providers covered by their health insurance. In countries where maternity services are provided by a national health service at low or no cost, such as Ireland and the UK, an obstetrician may be assigned to you. This is not to say you cannot change doctors if you want—you often can! If you are accessing private care through insurance or out of pocket, you may have the ability to "shop around" for who you feel is the best provider.

Alternatively, the classic midwifery model of care is based on the assumption that birth is a normal physiological process that most often leads to healthy outcomes for both moms and babies. The word "midwife" is the combination of the Middle English words "mid" (with) and "wife" (woman), whose literal meaning is *with woman.* Midwifery could arguably be one of the oldest support roles, and professions, within the human race—as we have always been having babies. Midwives are experts in supporting birth safely, they trust the labor process and are trained professionals who can assist with most emergencies, aside from surgery. A midwife may support births within the home but equally may work within a hospital or birth center. Although many people are unfamiliar with the midwifery model of care today, the truth is midwives existed long before obstetricians.

Research has shown that there are benefits to midwife-led care, especially when a person receives continuity of care from either one midwife or a team of midwives. Continuity of care means seeing the same person or group of people throughout pregnancy who will also be at your birth. A 2016 Cochrane Review showed that women accessing midwife-led care were less likely to experience interventions and were more likely to be satisfied with their care following birth.[3] The findings also showed women were less likely to have an epidural, receive an episiotomy and require an instrumental delivery via forceps or ventouse. Labor was more likely to start spontaneously, without the need for induction or artificial rupturing of membranes (releasing someone's waters). Other research suggests the risk of cesarean is reduced when this type of care is provided.[4] Overall, the midwife model of care is a safe option for those with uncomplicated pregnancies.

BIRTH CENTERS AND HOME BIRTH

Most people assume during pregnancy that they will give birth in a hospital. This will feel like the best place to birth for some, while others are seeking safe alternatives. A birth center may feel like a great "middle ground" for those who seek to step away from a hospital setting without necessarily birthing at home.

Birth centers are health facilities that may be alongside a hospital or freestanding. Both types are midwife-led, although a physician may oversee some practices. Birth centers are often home-like with less medical equipment and more items available to maximize comfort and promote the natural progression of labor. Many also feature pools for laboring and/or birth.

Recent research which took place in the United States looked at health outcomes for people with a higher BMI who accessed care in birth centers.[5] All of the expecting parents were "low-risk," meaning they had no known medical issues that would suggest complications were more likely. The study participants did not have an increase in prolonged labor, their waters being broken for more than twenty-four hours or postpartum hemorrhage. The health markers for their babies were also similar to the general population—meaning they did not have poorer outcomes. One of the most important results of this study reflects the difference in cesarean rates. Cesarean rates for plus size people are shockingly high in the United States, with rates fluctuating between 40-47%.[5] The birth center cesarean rate was markedly lower at 11.1%, with any necessary cesarean surgery being carried out in a hospital following transfer.[5] These lower cesarean rates may be attributed to the midwife model of care which aims to promote and protect the physiological process of birth. There was no significant increase in complications based on BMI in these facilities, making birth centers a safe choice for plus size people and their babies.

Home birth is another safe option for birthing families and no, you do not need to have an alternative lifestyle to find this path appealing. Findings from the UK Birthplace Study showed a significant decrease in interventions for "low-risk" parents, including those with a higher BMI, who chose to give birth at home.[6] A number of interventions were less likely, including: augmentation methods (Pitocin or syntocinon), pain relief in the form of an epidural or spinal analgesia, assisted delivery with forceps or ventouse, episiotomy and cesarean. First-time parents laboring at home were more likely to be transferred to a hospital and the most common reasons included: wanting more substantial pain relief (epidural), slow labor progression, meconium present in amniotic fluid and other signs that necessitated the use of continuous fetal monitoring. You will notice these common reasons are not emergency situations.

Although there has been an increasing interest in home birth, rates remain low in many countries. There are various reasons why people choose to birth at home, which may include:

- Wanting to birth in an environment that feels comfortable and safe— both physically and emotionally. You can customize your birth space more easily.
- Preparing for a more gentle birth experience. This may mean fewer interruptions, fewer people being present during labor, a dimly lit birth space, etc.
- Wanting to limit medical interventions. If an intervention becomes necessary, a trained midwife is there to provide support and help transfer to the nearest hospital if needed.
- A desire to labor or birth in water. Although many hospitals and birth centers now have pools, some may have restrictions that prevent them from being used by people of size. Such policies, which are influenced by weight stigma within maternity care, are not an issue when birthing at home.
- Seeking continuous one-to-one care with an experienced midwife or team of midwives. This type of care includes prenatal visits, birth support and postpartum follow-up.
- Some families would rather not travel during the height of labor to a hospital or birth center, which may be more of an issue if they live rurally.
- The ability to choose who will be present during birth. There are no imposed limits on birth support.
- Some families want to involve their older children in their birth or do

not have reliable child care options.
- Following birth, families can bond with their baby in their own space, which they may find more private and undisturbed. They can have visitors if and when desired, with no visiting hours to abide by.

There are different types of home birth that you will read about in the birth stories found in Part Two. The most common is an intentional, planned home birth which is attended by a midwife or duo of midwives. There are also really dramatic birth stories where babies are accidentally born at home, often called "born before arrival." An experience like this is usually the result of a baby making a speedy arrival—so quick in fact, there is not enough time to leave for the hospital or for midwives or paramedics to get to the house. The last type of home birth, and perhaps the most controversial, is freebirth. This is when a birth at home has been planned by expecting parents who wish to have no midwife, nurse or doctor present. They often trust the childbirth process and believe it should be undisturbed and instinctually driven. Many people who opt for freebirth have very personal reasons for doing so.

FINDING A SIZE-FRIENDLY PROVIDER

As you navigate your plus size pregnancy, one element worth considering is finding yourself a size-friendly provider. The last thing you or anyone else needs to experience while seeking maternity care is weight stigma or being mistreated because of your body size. Sadly, weight stigma felt by expecting parents has both physical and emotional implications for pregnancy and the postpartum period.[7] Finding a size-friendly provider is one way you can look after your health and advocate for yourself as you prepare for birth.

A size-friendly provider, sometimes referred to as fat-friendly, is someone who provides evidence-based, compassionate care which is individualized to your unique situation. They view you as a whole person and not just a BMI or number on a scale. You are not treated as a set of potential risks, but rather someone who can have a healthy, positive birth outcome. Size-friendly care is more holistic, extending beyond the scope of your BMI or body size, considering all aspects of your lifestyle.

A SIZE-FRIENDLY PROVIDER HAS THE FOLLOWING QUALITIES:

- Awareness of their own biases
- Provides compassionate support for people of all sizes and abilities
- Does not class you as "high-risk" solely based on your BMI
- Does not make assumptions about your eating habits and level of physical activity
- Has equipment suitable for use with people of size (blood pressure cuffs and speculums, for example)
- Treats you with dignity and respect
- Understands the importance of informed choice
- Acknowledges that you are the only expert of your body

FINDING THE RIGHT PRACTITIONER FOR YOU

There are multiple approaches to finding a size-friendly provider. One of the most valuable is asking other plus size parents, friends and family members for referrals. You may also be a member of a fat positive pregnancy or parenting group where you can ask for referrals in your area. If you are looking for a community to join, click over to the Fat and Pregnant website for information regarding online groups. Asking birth workers in your community is another great option. As a size-friendly doula and childbirth educator, I have experience supporting countless families and hearing a wide range of experiences, both positive and negative. Chances are the birth workers in your area also have some insight into who may or may not be size-friendly. Once you have created a list of providers, it's time to contact them.

WHAT TO ASK

Firstly, always inquire about their fees and if they are covered by your insurance, if that is needed. You may be able to interview some providers in person, while others are only available by phone or email. Unfortunately, some birth centers, midwives and facilities with pools for water birth may have BMI limitations. Asking about specific amenities is important, but also be mindful that it is oftentimes facility policies and not providers directly who make the call on what is available. It is also possible to advocate for change and the ability to labor in water even where limitations are set. Other questions you may want to ask include:

- What experience do they have in supporting people of size?
- Do they believe having a high BMI (with no underlying medical conditions) means someone's pregnancy is "high-risk?"
- What is their induction rate and under what circumstances might they suggest one?
- Under what circumstances may they suggest augmenting (speeding up) the labor process?
- What is their cesarean rate?
- What is their episiotomy rate?
- What is their philosophy regarding birth? *This is important because some providers see birth as more of a natural process that rarely needs intervention, while others are more likely to see birth as something that needs to be managed.*
- How do they feel about a birth plan?
- Are they the person who will be supporting you during labor? If not, who else may attend?
- What are their thoughts on doula support?
- Do they support freedom of movement during labor?
- What are their thoughts about you birthing in a variety of positions?
- Do they have any policies specifically for those with a higher BMI?

There are many other questions you could ask which may help you select the right provider. Explore what is important to you and begin there with your questions.

Always remember that you are the only person who knows which provider and place of birth feels right for you.

There are many pregnancy resources that suggest changing your current provider if you feel they are not the best person to support you. While this may be an option for some, it is also important to acknowledge that this is a privilege. Not everyone can afford a different provider and some insurance policies will only cover specific hospitals or provider types. Not everyone has access to transportation so they can seek care elsewhere. This is a complicated issue and exploring all of your options will provide the best picture of what is available for you specifically. In the case that you cannot switch providers or you are under a public healthcare system in which you cannot choose your care provider, hiring a birth doula may be another practical option for you.

Some doulas offer sliding fee scales and large doula associations often offer financial assistance programs for those in need. It is possible to have a positive birth experience even if your provider does not feel like the best fit. You may need to work with them by boosting your self advocacy skills, focusing more on setting healthy boundaries and ensuring you have support from family, friends and/or your partner. These topics are covered in Chapters Five and Six.

The Role of Childbirth Education

Childbirth education, also called prenatal education, was a social movement that began in the United States in the 1960s.[8] Parents and communities came together to promote more involvement and education within pregnancy care. This form of information sharing has continued to grow ever since across the globe. Classes that were once held in private homes and hospitals have now moved to a range of locations, including community centers, offices of midwives, doulas and online. The variety and type of classes have also diversified with more options for expecting parents of all types. The type of childbirth education available can now range from a short one-hour private session to twelve weeks of sessions within a group setting. As you explore your childbirth education options, you will quickly notice that not all programs are created equal and each has its own pros and cons.

Participation in childbirth education classes has gained in popularity, especially for first-time parents who may or may not have any particular fears or anxiety regarding the birth process. Such courses focus mainly on providing information about the stages of labor, pain relief options, emotional issues which may arise during labor and the early weeks of new parenting. Another important aim of prenatal preparation is promoting parents' confidence in the birth process, ensuring they feel powerful as they ask questions and make decisions. If courses are provided within group settings either online or in person, this creates another opportunity for continued social support both during pregnancy and following birth.

Birth preparation classes are often a component of routine prenatal care within high-income countries' healthcare systems, with classes commonly being offered within hospitals. They may also be provided routinely within public healthcare systems by midwives or other trained educators. While these classes have become common in some countries, others have not developed these programs as such and parents may have to rely on other resources to educate themselves or seek private childbirth education classes.

The content covered within childbirth education classes varies widely. Some may focus more heavily on how to have a healthy pregnancy and birth, while others focus primarily on the labor process itself. Programs may also promote a certain way to birth, such as The Bradley Method, whose classes are aimed at teaching techniques that will help expecting parents prepare for an unmedicated birth.[9] The Bradley Method website boasts that over 86% of families have had spontaneous, unmedicated vaginal births while using their methods. Lamaze International is another well-known prenatal education program, most commonly known for its breathing techniques, which teaches "six healthy birth practices."[10] These practices encourage parents to make informed choices, trust their body's natural ability to navigate labor and aim to reduce any unnecessary interventions. There are a large range of other specialized childbirth education classes, with some focusing on mindfulness and self-hypnosis.

Hypnobirthing is a method of pain management that can be used during labor and birth. This form of childbirth education involves using a mixture of visualization, relaxation and deep breathing techniques to help parents during labor. It is a complete program that aims to educate, inform and give expecting parents the tools they need to approach birth feeling calm and confident. The "hypno" part of hypnobirthing can immediately feel off-putting to some, but I like to remind people that hypnosis is nothing more than a naturally induced state of relaxed, focused concentration. Everyone experiences self-hypnotic states, for example when they are daydreaming. Hypnobirthing programs are beneficial for people from different backgrounds and those preparing for all types of birth. The tools and techniques backed by hypnobirthing programs increase emotional resilience, reduce levels of fear and stress, help buffer against stressful events, reduce the perception of pain and contribute to more positive birth experiences. One study which looked at the birth outcomes of parents who attended a hypnobirthing program found that they were better able to cope with the intensity of labor and were more likely to report that they had a positive birth experience. The study also indicated the following for parents who attended the hypnobirthing classes:[11]

- 23% increase in a spontaneous start to labor, versus an induction
- 14% reduction in instrumental delivery rates
- 30% reduction in epidural use
- 96% of participants went on to breastfeed their babies

Knowing the content covered within a prenatal program and the philosophy of the person conducting the class will help you decide if that form of education feels best for you. Higher quality childbirth education will go beyond surface level discussions and will include elements of informed decision-making, how to support hormones during labor, advocacy, cover a wide range of possible birth scenarios and will be unbiased in the information provided. Size-friendly prenatal education is free of weight bias and may also include information on common testing, challenges that may impact plus size pregnancy and tips for an easier birth experience. Classes held within hospital settings may provide a great overview of birth basics and give you an insight into the overall culture of birth within that facility. Do be mindful that some hospital-based classes are focused more on priming parents for giving birth within that facility and abiding by their protocols— essentially teaching you how to be a "good patient."

Debs Neiger is an independent midwife in the UK who has warned against childbirth education which she describes as "grooming for compliance."[12] This type of prenatal education prepares you for a role of compliance and portrays birth as working best when you do as you are told. It prepares expecting parents to leave their power and autonomy at the door, as it subtly plants the idea that birthing people are truly not in charge within the birth space. Below are some examples of the language which may be used and the beliefs often shared during childbirth education classes that "prepare" parents in this way.

- The use of language of allowance—"When you arrive at the hospital, we will do X."
- Ridiculing of physiological birth
- No consideration for birth center or home birth
- No consideration of birth without pain relief
- Many references that both doctors and midwives know best, as they are the experts
- Reassurance that interventions are never recommended without medical need
- Reassurance that any pain relief used has no implications for babies
- Some aspects of birth are inevitable
- Judgment toward those who make unconventional choices during pregnancy or birth
- Only basic information on labor and birth
- Conclude that other forms of childbirth education are pointless
- There is no need to create a birth plan

Childbirth education that grooms parents for compliance lacks discussion regarding autonomy, informed decision-making, confidence building and any reassurance that labor can be a positive, empowering experience. Birth is often depicted as something that parents just need to grit their teeth through and bear it to meet their baby on the other side. "All that matters is a healthy baby" is their tagline. More often than not such classes are offered within the very facilities that follow the medical model of maternity care. If you are hoping to avoid this type of prenatal education, the best way to gauge a potential class or program is to look through the topics covered and ensure they are centered around autonomy and choice.

A LOOK AT THE RESEARCH

Studies have indicated that childbirth education classes hold many benefits for expecting parents during both pregnancy and labor. With more pregnant people becoming fearful the childbirth process itself, there is a real place for prenatal programs to make a difference and assist parents in reducing their fears and anxiety levels. Approximately 20% of women living in developed countries experience high levels of childbirth fear, with another study indicating that 8% of first-time moms have a *severe* fear of childbirth.[13,14] It is important to know this information because expecting parents who are more fearful during pregnancy and the onset of labor are also more likely to have a challenging birth with higher intervention rates.[13] They are also more likely to have a cesarean birth.[13] Many studies have shown that first-time moms are more likely to have these fears and one study found that the more fearful first-time moms were during early labor, indicated as 3-5 cm dilated, the more pharmacological pain relief they used during the remainder.[15] When parents are more fearful of the childbirth process, this does impact the stress hormones that they release during labor. With an increase in adrenaline and norepinephrine, fearful birthing people are more likely to have a higher perception of pain, which increases their need for pain-relieving medication.

My belly grows more full of love with each passing day

Research has shown that childbirth education *does* impact expecting parents' fear and anxiety levels in a positive way. One form of childbirth education, called psycho-education was provided by midwives over the phone with expecting parents in Australia. The first-time moms experiencing this form of preparation were 11% more likely to have a vaginal birth and saw a 7% decrease in cesarean rates.[13] In Iran, which traditionally has not integrated birth preparation classes into their prenatal care, those who attended childbirth education classes regularly saw a reduction in anxiety, depression and fear levels during their pregnancy.[16] Parents were also more likely to have a positive birth experience and saw a reduction in postpartum depression scores.[17] Mindfulness-based prenatal classes have also proven to be beneficial, leading to lower rates of opioid analgesia use during labor and new parents had fewer symptoms of postpartum depression.[18]

Deciding where you would like to give birth, who will be supporting you and enrolling in size-friendly childbirth education are excellent ways to lay a solid foundation for your positive birth. No matter what stage of pregnancy you are in, whether you just got your positive test or your baby's estimated birth date is next week, it is never too late to make plans or changes. In the following chapters you will learn more about creating a birth plan, self advocacy, how to work with your hormones during labor and ways your birth partner can support you on the big day.

Chapter Five:
CREATING A BIRTH PLAN
THAT WORKS FOR YOU

A birth plan is a document that is created by expecting parents, outlining what their wishes are for birth and what is important to them. It may be written, printed and given to a healthcare professional weeks or months before birth takes place. This is an excellent way to create meaningful dialogue and also gauge your provider's reaction. If they are unwilling to discuss your wishes or are shooting down everything you have included, that may be a clear indication that your healthcare provider's philosophy regarding birth does not match your own.

This is also another way to uncover the belief systems regarding intervention where you opt to give birth. "This is the way things are done here," is often a pretext for care that is not evidence-based and may imply a sense of rigidity from your provider. Hopefully you are met with enthusiasm and support from your chosen provider, who may also have questions for clarification on how they can accommodate you best. If you are met with a lack of enthusiasm or worse, contempt, you will need to decide how best to proceed. You could continue on with that provider, now knowing you may need to ramp up your advocacy efforts or find additional support, like a doula. Alternatively, finding another provider or facility to birth at may be preferable. You can see why it may be better to introduce your birth plan to your provider ahead of time.

A birth plan essentially is a tool that helps you communicate with whoever will be supporting you during birth. It may be created for birth of all types, including spontaneous start of labor, induction of labor, planned and unplanned cesarean. No matter what way you choose or need to give birth, every parent on the planet has at least *one thing* that is important to them aside from the survival of both themselves and their baby.

One English survey indicated that more than 35% of parents begin thinking about the type of birth they want even before they conceive.[1] A document like a birth plan not only helps facilitate communication, it will also encourage you and your birth partner to educate yourselves and consider all of your options for labor and birth. Many expecting parents do not realize the true breadth of decision-making that is upon them until they start digging into the stages of labor, what may happen and the different types of interventions which may be suggested. This prenatal learning, which may be undertaken by yourself or with the help of a childbirth educator, will help direct you in discovering what is important to *you*— which may not reflect what is important to someone else, and that is okay. It sounds cliché, but knowledge is power in the birth space. Going through the process of creating a birth plan and being aware of your options will increase your knowledge and ability to assist in making informed choices. Bashi Hazard, a lawyer and director of Human Rights in Childbirth, believes a birth plan is "the closest expression of informed consent that a woman can offer her caregiver prior to commencing labor." [2]

The culture surrounding birth often discourages the creation of birth plans, sometimes called birth preferences. One busy maternity hospital in Dublin, Ireland went so far as to post signs in their bathrooms that explicitly stated, "It is not necessary for you to write a birth plan." Some people oppose their creation on the basis that experts in birth should be trusted to have the best interests of both birthing people and their babies in mind. What this neglects to acknowledge is how provider attitudes, belief systems, fear of litigation and the culture in which they work impacts the care they provide. This also fails to address how weight stigma has led to compounded interventions for fat folks within the birth space.

Expecting parents across the globe are also frequently told that birth is unpredictable anyway so there is no point in creating a list of preferences that are unlikely to take place. This story is pitched as a false sense of protection—"Don't get your hopes up and you can't be disappointed." What this narrative is *really doing*, along with the "all that matters is a healthy baby" line, is encouraging parents to be as small, accommodating and silent as possible. This benefits medical professionals and creates fewer waves in a healthcare system that values compliance.

MICHELLE MAYEFSKE

THE DANGERS OF "GOING WITH THE FLOW"

Many expecting parents are recommended to take a more "hands off" approach during labor, simply being urged to "go with the flow" while casting their birth plan aside. One must consider—exactly whose flow are you going with? Are you going with the flow of the hospital setting? Are you going with the flow of your provider's belief system, staying within the parameters they have chosen as appropriate? Bashi Hazard explains the reality of "going with the flow" within institutionalized maternity care. Even if you do not create a written birth plan yourself, "There *is* a birth plan—one driven purely by care providers and hospital protocols..." (original emphasis)[2] When we consider that high tech modern maternity care is often characterized as risk-based and medicalized, "going with the flow" often means signing yourself up for an experience which will involve interventions being recommended on a routine basis versus necessitated by medical need—"too much too soon."

Many people who view their future birth through the lens of the *fearful fat* narrative may accept their body as incapable—there is something "wrong" with them. These expecting parents often enter the maternity system with an already deep lack of confidence in their body's ability. If this is reflected back to them by their provider, feelings of mistrust and alienation from their own body may be amplified. Weight biased healthcare professionals create their own "flow" of normality and are quick to apply more high-intervention strategies if they view fat birth from a place of fear and risk versus a normal life event taking place within a bigger body. Research has shown that obstetric nurses who view birth as more "risky" are more likely to recommend interventions, including continuous electronic fetal monitoring and epidural use, both of which have further potential risks.[3]

Today's maternity culture, which pathologizes fatness, is also quick to blame plus size pregnant bodies for any complications, thus proving to expecting parents that they were right all along—their fat body truly is incapable. Rather than shining the light on themselves and blaming weight discrimination for intensely interventionist care, the default has become pinning all responsibility on fat bodies themselves. If a fat person does have a challenging birth, theirs is used as a "cautionary tale," repeated to expecting parents as a warning to do as they are told.

INFORMED CHOICE

There has been much discussion within the birth world surrounding "informed consent," a term which I and many other birth professionals have abandoned in recent years in exchange for "informed choice." The words "informed consent" within the medical community imply that consent will eventually be given or is the end goal, which should never be the aim of truly informed choice. Informed choice is when you are given options to choose from in regards to treatments, tests, monitoring and procedures. You are given the full details of the proposed action, its potential benefits, potential risks, alternatives and the expected outcome. This information is presented to you in an unbiased way so you can decide which action feels best for your unique situation.

Informed choice within maternity care is not an assumed given. Some professionals feel it is *their responsibility* to provide all of the facts so parents can decide what feels best, however, this is countered by other professionals who feel it is up to the *parents themselves* to both find and ask for information. This has proven to be incredibly problematic when higher rates of intervention are the norm. One English survey found that 67% of expecting parents were not told by healthcare professionals that they had the right to decline interventions.[1] The results of another study showed that more than 26% of new parents experienced informal coercion during their childbirth.[4] These parents felt pressured by healthcare providers to agree to interventions and were more likely to experience coercive practices if they had a cesarean or instrumental vaginal birth.

Worryingly, there are additional barriers to informed choice being the norm within maternity care today. Both midwives and doctors cite they simply do not have the time for discussions with parents about decision-making.[5] Expecting parents echoed this issue of time constraints during a study in Wales, stating they wanted to discuss their options but felt their provider was too busy to do so.[5] They self-limited the questions they asked in response to this. Providers also indicated that their fear of future litigation was a prominent concern and a driving force for their recommendations of intervention and thus, often not medically necessary.[5] This fear of litigation comes up time and time again in the research surrounding high intervention rates in hospital settings. Healthcare providers further admitted to using coercion and risk-based language as a measure to steer expecting parents down a path that they felt was "right" and would protect them from potential litigation.[5] One registrar interviewed said the following when discussing an expecting parent's choices regarding the birth of their baby in a breech position:

> Giving them a choice is not enough. They need to know the reality behind it [vaginal breech delivery] . . . about the head getting stuck definitely. You can give them scare stories but you don't even have to do that. You just have to mention a complication. Something like the baby might die. . .[5]

Doctors especially knew how to frame information so expecting parents would either feel like they had no choice or the best one was that which the doctor had suggested. This is *not* informed choice and these coercive tactics continue to uphold high intervention rates and create the potential for further harm to moms and babies.

A lack of informed choice may present in numerous ways, such as:

- A provider only presenting the information that will convince you to agree with them.
- Presenting only *part* of the information needed to make an informed choice.
- Interventions are suggested but the option *to do nothing* is not mentioned.
- Assumed compliance—usually paired with language of allowance, such as, "Hop up on the bed there and I'll check your cervix," or "I'm just going to break your waters now."

Coercion may also look like misinformation or being completely lied to. My jaw dropped when I attended a client's labor which was leading toward a forceps-assisted birth. As the doctor prepared the forceps, he said to my client, "Don't worry, this cannot hurt your baby," which was a blatant lie. Anyone who researches the potential risks of forceps knows they can cause facial lacerations, injury to the eyes, facial palsy (muscle weakness in the face), skull fractures and more. Lying to parents is *not* doing them a favor or protecting them—it can lead to further trauma and dehumanizes them as nothing more than a vessel.

Knowing that a provider may not give you accurate information or all of the information you need creates a climate of mistrust, leaving many parents asking, "Am I getting the right information?" or "Is this really being suggested because it is in the best interest of me and my baby?" It has caused skepticism within the birth space, with expecting parents questioning whether labor interventions are being suggested out of convenience, due to fears of litigation or if recommendations are truly medically necessary. As you can imagine, this is a complex issue and not all providers want to be painted with the same brush. There *are* many wonderful maternity care providers who ensure pregnant people are the fully-informed, key decision-makers of their own care. However, we cannot ignore the fact that the entire obstetric world functions within a patriarchal system that endorses a lack of informed choice for women.

You have the right to ask questions during your pregnancy, as you create your birth plan and during labor. It may be helpful to create a list of questions for future prenatal visits. A list will not only help you remember, but it will also create a space for dialogue during your appointment—"I've brought some questions with me today that I would like to discuss."

The decisions I make are meaningful for me and my baby

The Language of Risk

Dr Sara Wickham has done amazing work surrounding the high levels of risk-based language used within maternity care. She states, "In modern midwifery and medical practice, risk-related words abound. There's high-risk, low-risk, increased risk and relative risk; risk analysis, risk management, risk factors and risk assessment."[6] There are downsides to always using this risk-heavy language. The word "risk" itself tends to invoke feelings of fear, even if the word is used to denote a decrease, such as "reduction in risk." It may also exaggerate any potential downside, ranging from being simply unhelpful to misleading for expecting parents. Furthermore, the word "risk" is never entirely eliminated from modern classification systems used to label expecting parents as either "high-risk" or "low-risk". Both imply there is some sense of danger surrounding the pregnant body and birth. This can be especially problematic if plus size pregnancies are automatically classified as "high-risk" based on BMI alone.

Much of the other language used within maternity care is focused around what is viewed as "abnormal," and as such, Wickham goes on to state, "Western medicine has been so focused on defining what is pathological that there are few terms and expressions that tell a woman how marvelously capable her body is..."[6]

The focus of pregnancy often tends to be on what can possibly go wrong, completely missing the mark on how so many things *can go right.* Instead of continuing this risk-based and fear-focused language, Wickham recommends replacing the word "risk" with "chance" in as many instances as possible.[7] So instead of saying, "You are at a higher risk of developing gestational diabetes," a provider could state the alternative, "You have an increased chance of developing gestational diabetes." These sentences are giving the same information, just in a different way that does not revolve around risk-talk. It would be wonderful to see a change in language use by birth workers and expecting parents alike to help reduce the culture of fear around pregnancy and birth.

RELATIVE RISK AND ABSOLUTE RISK

These are two terms worth knowing, as they may impact your informed decision-making process as you prepare your birth plan and journey through pregnancy. A relative risk is when one rate is compared to another rate, such as this statement on racial disparities in US maternity care— "Black women are three times more likely to die from a pregnancy-related cause than White women."[8]

Notice that this fact is comparing deaths between two groups of people, however, it does not indicate the actual rate of death for either group. When only a relative risk is provided, the actual risk(s) are missing. Furthermore, being given a relative risk provides no other details, like *why* these racial disparities exist or what action can be taken to support Black expecting parents.

When relative risk is referenced within maternity care for people of size, it is usually comparing rates of someone with a lower BMI to someone with a higher BMI. An *actual risk* tells you the actual statistical likelihood for someone who is your size, age, race etc. without comparing one group to another. This is important information because the likelihood of developing certain pregnancy conditions can be presented in different ways, depending on whether the relative risk, absolute risk or both are provided.

A great example that will help distinguish the two is the case for developing gestational diabetes. Many fat folks are told they are "three times more likely to develop gestational diabetes" because of their size. This is the *relative risk*. Again, notice how the relative risk does not indicate what two rates are being compared. You are not getting the full breadth of information when only the relative risk is provided. "Three times more likely" may also sound very frightening if you do not know the actual likelihood of you developing gestational diabetes or any other condition for that matter!

The *actual risk* would sound more like this—"You have a 20% chance of developing gestational diabetes." You are getting the detailed statistical likelihood when the actual risk is referenced. Twenty percent may still feel like a lot to some people, but it also means there is an 80% likelihood that you will *not* develop gestational diabetes! Here are the absolute risks of developing gestational diabetes from one study, broken down by BMI categories.[9] I have to say it—keep in mind BMI is a flawed classification system in and of itself and the study participants were divided into groups with no regards to other health markers.

- BMI 25 to <30: 6.74%
- BMI 30 to <35: 13.42%
- BMI 35 to <40: 12.79%
- BMI ≥40: 20%

Knowing the difference between relative risk and absolute risk can assist with making decisions both during pregnancy and labor. As you create your birth plan, consider where you will be giving birth, who will be supporting you and what is important to you. You are the boss of your body and your birth, making you the key decision-maker no matter what path labor may take. Every person's birth plan is unique to them and some people may feel very strongly about what they want, while others are a bit more laid back. You know your personality and what feels best for you.

TIPS FOR CREATING A BIRTH PLAN

KNOWLEDGE IS POWER

Remember *why* you are creating a birth plan. Your list of preferences is not a contract or a guarantee, but a useful way to learn all of your options and communicate them effectively with your care provider. Your birth plan is a massive step in ensuring your voice is *heard* within the birth space. Your unique needs matter and you are worthy of respectful, dignified care at any size and no matter your health status. Creating a birth plan with your birth partner ensures you are on the same page and they are better able to assist with advocacy on the day. Use your knowledge gained to positively impact your pregnancy, promote more agency over your experience and help gauge whether your provider is the best fit for you.

FOCUS ON YOU

What birth experience are you truly hoping and preparing for? You may find that your choices are not common or part of the "usual protocol" wherever you intend to give birth. This is okay and your preferences still matter. You are the only person giving birth to your baby and as such, your voice should be heard the loudest.

PLAN B, C AND D

When first creating your birth plan, your plan A is what your ideal birth would look like, including every detail that is important to you. Do consider alternatives and go over various scenarios with your birth partner and provider, if you wish, so you are better prepared for any path labor may take. If a cesarean is something you are hoping to avoid, including birth preferences in the event that it becomes necessary is still important. "In Case of Cesarean" is a common heading I encourage clients to include at the bottom of their birth plan. All parents still have things which are important to them if a surgical birth becomes a reality, which may include optimal cord clamping, skin to skin, lowering of the drapes during birth and more.

STOP "ALL OR NOTHING" THINKING

Many parents will say there was a time during their birth when "the birth plan went out the window." What they are usually referring to is when things began feeling out of control and consent became patchy. This may also be said in relation to experiencing the cascade of interventions— when one intervention led to another and parents began feeling like none of their wishes were being considered any longer. The reality is that in the vast majority of cases, even when one item on a birth plan is not fulfilled, many other elements are still a possibility. These include optimal cord clamping, skin to skin following birth, announcing of the baby's sex and more. If it becomes necessary to side step your birth plan in any way, even more than once, that does *not* mean your ability to make informed choices or have the rest of your birth plan adhered to has come to a dead end.

DO NOT FORGET THE GOLDEN HOUR

The "golden hour" is considered the first hour immediately following birth. This is a special time when new parents have an opportunity to bond with their baby, initiate breastfeeding and there are so many benefits to having baby skin to skin. Placing baby directly on your bare chest helps regulate their body temperature and blood sugar levels, regulates their heart rate and breathing, promotes colonization of your baby's microbiome (which builds their immune system), reduces stress hormone production (namely cortisol) and stimulates the release of hormones which promote breastfeeding and early bonding with both parents.[10] The benefits continue for babies who are born preterm, with skin to skin contact improving blood flow to the brain, promoting growth, improved nervous system functioning and more stable sleep patterns.[11] As you consider your options for the moments directly following birth, you may wish to state your preferences regarding a managed or physiological birth of your placenta, the initial neonatal check, vaccinations, vernix, erythromycin eye drops (which are common in the United States) and what you would like done with your placenta—as some parents like to keep it for cultural reasons or placenta encapsulation.

TOPICS TO CONSIDER

So what exactly is there to think about? Many parents break down their birth plan into stages—something along the lines of "admissions, labor, birth, newborn care, in case of cesarean". This does make it clearer and easier to read for both your care provider and your birth partner if they need to refer to it during labor.

The main topics usually considered are in relation to the augmentation (speeding up) of labor, types of fetal monitoring, the frequency of internal vaginal exams, your feelings on pain management, movement during labor, which way you would like to push—including position and coached versus spontaneous pushing—and those initial moments following birth. If you are having an induction of labor, you may also include more detail regarding the pace at which you would like the steps of labor induction performed. For example, if your hospital has a policy states that Pitocin should be administered in conjunction with the releasing of your waters once you are 2 cm dilated, you may prefer to opt-out of using Pitocin immediately to see if labor begins on its own. Some people make this choice if they are hoping to postpone or completely avoid the use of Pitocin. They may choose to wait and see if their body will create contractions on its own without its administration. This preference could be included within your birth plan and of course discussed on the day.

HOW TO USE YOUR BRAIN

The BRAIN acronym is an amazing tool to assist you in creating your birth plan and making informed decisions during pregnancy, labor and as a parent more generally. It really is something that should be taught to school children and adults everywhere, as BRAIN can be used in literally *any situation* where you need to make a decision. If a test, treatment or procedure is recommended for you or your baby during pregnancy or birth, consider these things:

Benefits

What are the potential benefits for you, your baby and your family? Are the benefits going to last in the short term or long term? How likely are you to experience the potential benefits? If statistics are referenced ("One-in-four moms…"), are they evidence-based—meaning, is it supported by research? Weigh the possible benefits up with the potential risks and alternatives, outlined below.

Risks

What are the potential risks for you, your baby and your family? These risks are not guarantees, but they are a possibility. May the potential risks last short term or long term? If a provider says there are increased risks because of your weight or BMI, is there evidence to support it? When potential risks are presented, are they relative or absolute risks?

Alternatives

What are the alternatives to whatever is being suggested? Sometimes an alternative may be a different intervention or simply doing nothing! There are *always* alternatives, and some may appeal to you while others do not. You can go one step further with alternatives and start the BRAIN process again. Once you review your initial option and identify possible alternatives, you can begin looking at the potential pros, cons and alternatives *to that alternative* as well. Stay with me—I promise to provide a clear example.

Intuition

What is your intuition telling you? This aspect of our mind and body seems to be stomped out of us very early on. Ever heard "trust your gut?" That is your intuition talking, my friend, and it is not unusual or problematic if you lean into that feeling every now and again. Pregnancy is the perfect time to slow down if you can, quiet your busy mind and reconnect with your body. Everyone feels differently of course but I have met many parents who said their own intuition had a bit of a rebirth, a rising up from the ashes, when they conceived. Many moms-to-be will say they *just knew* they were pregnant within days of actual conception or they predicted the sex of their baby based mostly on an instinctual knowing. Birth can be intuitive, instinctual and empowering too.

If your intuition is not bubbling over, steering you in the right direction *for you*, that may be an indicator that you simply need more information, support or time to help you decide.

Now or Nothing

"N" can stand for either "now" or "nothing." Firstly, do you need to make a decision *right now* or do you have time? In most cases, even in a busy birth space, you do have time to discuss things—even if it is seconds or a few minutes. Creating a gap where you can ask questions, gather more information and *take a breath* will allow you to make a truly informed choice. You may assert yourself if time allows by saying, "We would like five minutes to talk in private and decide," "Can you tell me more about that, including the possible benefits and risks?" or "We would like to revisit that option in an hour," for example.

"Nothing" is just as it sounds—what happens if you decide to do nothing and continue as you are? And here you begin the BRAIN loop again—what are the potential benefits and risks of doing nothing?

BRAIN IN ACTION

Example: Your baby's estimated birth date is tomorrow and your provider offers you a membrane sweep. You are 1cm dilated, your cervix is effaced 25% and soft.

A membrane sweep, sometimes called membrane stripping, is often suggested as part of an internal vaginal exam during the last weeks of pregnancy. Membrane sweeping is a form of labor induction and as such, *should be discussed* prior to being done. The process involves your care provider inserting a finger into the vaginal cavity and up to the cervix. The cervix must be dilated at least 1cm for the sweep to take place. Your provider's finger is then inserted into and just past the cervix, at the very base of the womb. Here, a rotating "sweep" motion is done with the finger, separating the base of the amniotic sac that your baby is in with the bottom of the uterus. It is believed that this procedure increases prostaglandin hormone levels, which can help tip the body into starting labor. Why have I shared all of this information with you?—because knowing what a procedure physically entails is a critical part of informed decision-making.

Potential Benefits:

The membrane sweep could help start labor. If a medical induction is being recommended, a membrane sweep may also help you avoid one. If your membrane sweep is done at forty-one weeks of pregnancy, a sweep will reduce the likelihood of you progressing to forty-two weeks pregnant by half.[12]

Potential Risks:

Anytime anything enters the vagina, there is potential for bacteria to be brought into the body. Higher levels of internal vaginal exams are linked to increased infection risk.[13] You must be at least one centimeter dilated and the procedure itself is classed as "painful" by 70% of expecting moms.[14] Chances are it will not be effective. One in eight women will go into labor if a membrane sweep is performed at forty weeks of pregnancy.[12] Nine percent of membrane sweeps result in artificial releasing of amniotic fluid.[15] This can lead to a longer labor and formal medical induction of labor if your body does not begin creating contractions on its own. Knowing this information may influence if and *when* you consent to a sweep, if desired. Membrane sweeps can cause spotting and uterus irritability, leading to contractions that come and go in an erratic way.[12] This may not bother some parents, but it may lead to increased feelings of anxiety if someone feels unsure about whether labor is starting or not.

Alternatives:

Alternatives include: declining a membrane sweep so spontaneous labor may begin, delaying a membrane sweep until a later date or opting for an induction of labor. If a membrane sweep is offered before your baby's estimated birth date and there is no medical need to start labor *now,* waiting until labor begins is absolutely reasonable. Four percent of people will give birth on their baby's estimated birth date and 70% will give birth within ten days of their "due date."[16] If you decide to wait for labor to begin and change your mind later, you can always request a sweep!

And lastly, if labor just is not starting and you feel ready to begin the labor process with some help, a medical induction can be arranged. When you consider all possible alternatives, you can then use BRAIN to assess those options, too. In this case, an alternative to a membrane sweep is a medical induction. You can then use BRAIN to discover what the potential benefits, risks and more are for induction. BRAIN is all about digging that bit deeper so you get a full picture of what your options are so you feel more confident making the decision that feels right for you.

Intuition:

What is your **intuition** telling you? During my second pregnancy I was offered a membrane sweep. I did not want one because I knew why my body had not gone into labor—my mom was on vacation in Hawaii. I *just knew* my body would relax and labor would start once she returned home from her trip. Four hours after my mom's plane landed, when I was forty weeks and five days pregnant, I went into labor. Coincidence? I did not think so.

Now or Nothing:

A membrane sweep is not something you have to decide on **now.** It is not an emergency, so you have time to think. You can take a few minutes to decide if you are actually at a prenatal visit when one is suggested or have time to think about it as you wait for your next visit with your provider.

This is one example of informed decision-making during late pregnancy. BRAIN may not be as easily recalled if you have entered a more challenging stage of labor and need to focus on getting through each contraction. This is why ensuring your birth partner knows this acronym is critical, so they may advocate on your behalf and ask questions that will assist in decision-making if an intervention is recommended.

The Cascade of Interventions

When using the BRAIN method, another phenomenon to consider is what is referred to as the "cascade of interventions," sometimes called the "carousel of interventions." Both refer to circumstances in which one intervention is more likely to lead to another and another.

Oftentimes when parents agree to an intervention, they may not consider the path that choice may be leading them down in terms of further interventions. Many of the current interventions available, including Pitocin to speed up labor and forms of pain relief, do have implications for the body's normal production of hormones throughout the labor and birth process. Dr Sarah Buckley is an expert in the field of hormones during labor. She has contributed to numerous publications and described how disruptions in hormones may be amplified when one intervention leads to another. Further interventions are often required during labor to help manage, prevent or treat side effects that may present following the original intervention. For example: if a birthing person consents to an epidural, this often leads to a reduction in oxytocin levels. To compensate for this and increase the speed of labor, synthetic oxytocin (Pitocin or syntocinon) may be administered. Prolonged use of Pitocin has the ability to desensitize maternal oxytocin receptors, which in turn increases the risk of postpartum hemorrhage.[17] This is the hormonal ripple effect one intervention may have for the rest of labor.

The cascade of interventions must not only be seen through the lens of hormone production. That is of course a big piece, but it is not the only aspect to consider. For example, if using the BRAIN method when deciding to opt for an epidural or not, one potential risk is associated with the numbing sensation that is standard with this form of pain relief and felt from the waist down. The implications of this numbing may lead to further interventions if a laboring person cannot feel when and how to push once they are fully dilated. If an individual is struggling to feel this sensation, further interventions, including an episiotomy to widen the vaginal opening, and the risk of instrumental birth (via forceps or vacuum delivery) are increased. It is worth noting that further interventions may not become a reality at all, but in order to make a fully-informed choice, the possibility of further interventions and what those may mean for you and your baby must be considered.

SELF ADVOCACY

It is all well and good to create a birth plan and become knowledgeable about childbirth, but if you do not know how to advocate for yourself, your birth preferences will either remain in your head or on paper, never to be realized. Throughout this text I have highlighted time and again that *you* are in charge of your body, your baby and your experience. You are the only expert of your body, your needs and how you can best be supported. I have given you both information and tools to help you identify what feels right for you. Now it is your turn to take the fruits of your exploration and *make what matters to you known*. If you want particular support during your pregnancy and birth, you actually *need to tell people* what you need. No one is a mind reader and in the world of medicalized birth, if you do not advocate for yourself, others may assume you are ready and willing to "go with the flow" of standard maternity care.

Self advocacy is the ability to represent yourself in articulating your own needs. It includes knowing and understanding your rights, including the right to bodily autonomy in birth, and making informed decisions so you can access the care and support you need. In the birth world, self advocacy ensures that *you and your unique wishes* are at the center of your care and not pushed aside or forgotten. Self advocacy can feel like a scary thing to do within a culture that encourages maternal figures to *always put themselves last.* Your voice may need to be even louder and more assertive if you want to ensure it is heard within the busy world of birth. The following are the keys to assertiveness in maternity care:

- **Know Your Rights:** Be clear with yourself and others that you have the legal right to be the central decision-maker in your maternity care. You are worthy of dignity and respectful care and having the full scope of information to support you in decision-making. If your rights are not being respected or you are receiving inadequate care, you have the option to make a formal complaint and access support services.
- **Know What You Want and Why:** Being knowledgeable about your options will help build your confidence when speaking about the care you want. Be clear and unapologetic when you describe what is important to you and how you want certain aspects of your care facilitated. You can still remain flexible while creating a birth plan and sharing that with your care provider. Knowing the different paths labor may take and how your priorities might shift is key.
- **Take Up Space:** You are the most important person when it comes to your care and it is time you start acting like it! Developing your confidence may take time but it will be felt by those around when you enter a space with strength versus timidity. Consider what you would like to say before you meet with a care provider, bring a list of questions you have prepared, practice what you will say if you need to and consider your body language when you are around others. You are not wasting someone's time by indicating your wishes.
- **Choose Your Support Team:** It is easier to assert yourself when you know you have the support of others who are on the same page and willing to advocate for you if necessary. Ensure your birth partner is up to speed with your wishes and they are clear on how to support you during labor with confidence. If you are looking for additional support, a doula is another option. Having a size-friendly provider can be another critical component to your care.
- **Have an Exit Strategy:** If you are not receiving the respectful, holistic

care that you deserve which is free of weight stigma, it may be possible to seek care elsewhere. You may be able to switch doctors, find a midwife, opt for a home birth or find another facility.

- **Setting Boundaries:** Creating healthy boundaries with your provider has many benefits. It can help reduce stress, increase your self-esteem, promote feelings of understanding and help develop stronger communication. Everyone can benefit from boundary setting, however, it may be particularly useful for those who have a hard time making decisions, may feel guilty when they say "no," or have a history of making sacrifices for others at their own expense. You may be able to set boundaries before even meeting with a provider when you contact them initially to see if they are size-friendly. Alternatively, you may set some boundaries during a booking appointment, within new client paperwork, send a letter before an upcoming appointment or during any appointment you may have. "No mention of BMI or weight but happy to discuss diet, physical activity and general wellness," is a boundary many parents of size may set with their provider to ensure the focus of their care is not constantly revolving around their weight.
- **Learn How to Say "No":** This is one of the topics expecting parents struggle with most. They may want to decline a test, monitoring or procedure but may not know how to do so. Discomfort in saying no often stems from one's own beliefs surrounding compliance and "letting someone down" by not agreeing with them. There are many ways to opt-out of anything in the birth space with language varying on the spectrum of assertiveness. Practice phrases, such as "We'd like more time to consider that before making a decision," "I'm not sure how I feel about that, can you give me more information?", "I'm saying 'no' now but would like to revisit this in an hour," "I'm not consenting to that," "Please respect my no," "Stop what you are doing NOW!" If you feel like you are being coerced or bullied into making a decision, tell your care provider this. Saying "no" does not give providers the green light to continue trying to change your mind. If you are firm on your decision, make that known—"I am not changing my mind about this" or "I have already given you my answer."

FAT BIRTH

Chapter Six:
KICKASS BIRTH SUPPORT

Who you decide to have as your birth partner during labor is another important decision. Some people value having fewer people in their birth space, while others want a collection of family and friends along with their intimate partner. What I do urge you to consider is how the people you invite to your birth may impact it. What energy are they going to bring? Are they great at navigating highly emotive experiences or are they a bundle of nerves? Are they going to take a more active role or sit back as a spectator?—and how do *you* feel about that? It is also important to consider that you may not know how they will react until the actual day—and how do *you* feel about that? You may find that this aspect of birth preparation involves a lot of exploration and frank internal dialogue.

You do not "owe" anyone attendance at your birth—not your mother, not your sister, not your friend, your partner's family or anyone else. The labor process is a very intimate, vulnerable time and you are going to experience things you never have before. Your body will also go through a gamut of bodily functions, which may include: coughing, sneezing, sweating, crying, peeing, farting, vomiting, pooping and, yes, some people even orgasm. Think about who will add to your experience without judgment. This is not a time to put other people's feelings above your own—yours matter the most and if the wrong person is in your birth space, there are consequences. At the very least, they may make you feel awkward, self-conscious or embarrassed. Worst-case scenario—if they are anxious, fearful or they keep trying to jump in and "rescue you," they can unintentionally disrupt the labor process. This may impact your ability to focus, vocalize as you need to, move as you want to, indicate what your needs are and increase stress hormones, like adrenaline. Stress hormones reduce the production of oxytocin, the very hormone that keeps labor moving! A sudden increase in adrenaline levels can *slow* labor by making contractions further apart, weaker and less effective. For you, this may mean an increase in pain perception and a more drawn-out labor—both of which increase the likelihood of interventions for you and your baby.

Choosing who you want at your birth is the first step—preparing them is another. Creating boundaries can help you both feel more confident and prepared for the day. For example, if your mom is going to be supporting you, start with when you want her to join you. At home? The hospital or birth center? You may indicate some other preferences you have—how you feel about touch, if you want her notifying others about your labor progress (I had a friend whose mom was sharing her cervical dilation *in real-time* on social media *without her knowledge!)*, where you want her while you are pushing, etc. You also have the right to ask anyone to leave. If someone is violating boundaries or is simply losing their shit watching you labor, you can absolutely change your plans. If your stomach just dropped at the thought of doing this, then you may need to rely on your partner, midwife, nurse or someone else to help facilitate it. In fact, I encourage you to do so. Have an exit strategy prepared in case it becomes necessary and tell people that if they are asked to leave, they *need* to respect that decision.

No matter who you chose to have at your birth *do not underestimate how incredible they can be on the day!* Women who receive loving support are more likely to reflect positively on their birth.[1] A birth partner is someone who is there to support you physically and emotionally. While many people have their intimate partner attend their birth, there are of course circumstances when the birth partner is someone else, like a family member, friend or professional doula. Whomever is at your labor, they may also help with the practical aspects of birth and use their voice to help advocate on your behalf. Sometimes birth partners may feel like they are the least knowledgeable person in the room, so they may unintentionally shrink into the background. The reality is that while they may not have any medical expertise, they are the only person in the room who knows you best. They know your strengths and your areas of vulnerability. Their more intimate knowledge of you makes them the best person to create and protect your oxytocin bubble of safety.

OXYTOCIN- YOUR TICKET TO LABOR LAND

Oxytocin is often called the "love hormone," as it is the hormone of connection and trust. Our bodies release oxytocin whenever we do "feel good" things: laugh, eat delicious food, listen to music, dance, meditate, hug, have sex, orgasm and the peak oxytocin experience is when we give birth. As pregnancy advances, the level of oxytocin within the body increases and the uterus begins to have more oxytocin receptor cells.[2] This increase helps the cervix soften in preparation for labor and ensures contractions are more effective.

This wonderfully intoxicating hormone is made by the hypothalamus and stored in the pituitary gland. It is pumped into the bloodstream via pulses to help with labor progression. When your baby's head puts pressure on the cervix, this not only helps with dilation, it keeps the positive oxytocin loop going. Oxytocin *decreases* cortisol levels, which has a calming effect and can lead to both lower blood pressure and heart rate. It is your best friend during birth, as it helps activate your parasympathetic nervous system, triggering some great natural pain-relieving properties.[2] Oxytocin reaches its highest peak within the first hour following birth. If a new parent is doing skin to skin, this hormone is what helps warm their newborn, helps the uterus contract to prevent postpartum bleeding, facilitates bonding and is a key ingredient in breastfeeding.[2] Oxytocin is just one hormone within an intricate system that works together to promote labor as a safe, efficient and calm experience.

Your birth partner's key role in supporting you is to keep the oxytocin train moving. There are many ways they can facilitate this and it all begins during pregnancy. Labor is not the time for discovery—both you and your birth partner should be setting the stage for optimal oxytocin release long before you feel the first twinges of labor. Throughout pregnancy you are ultimately creating a climate of trust. As the birthing person, you are learning to trust the labor process and your body. You are letting go of any preconceived ideas and any limitations you may have reserved for yourself. You are learning to trust that your birth partner knows what to do and that you can rely on them, no matter what path labor takes. Your birth partner is not only learning the basics of birth and how to support you, they are learning to trust that you will indicate your needs as they arise. They also begin to trust *themselves*—that they have put in the work to be the best birth support that they can be.

I trust my birth partner to create and protect my safe space for birth

PROMOTING OXYTOCIN

Supporting your hormones during birth is a two-way street. On one hand, you want to help promote oxytocin to keep labor moving—and on the other, you want to reduce any sudden increases in stress hormones that can hinder labor progression. Think of oxytocin like the accelerator in a car and stress hormones as the brakes.

Our bodies and hormone systems have evolved over millions of years to assist with sustaining pregnancy, birth and postpartum bonding.[2] Your body *wants* to birth in a calm, private environment and keep both you and your baby safe. If you become fearful, stressed or anxious during labor, your body will begin to create higher levels of adrenaline and norepinephrine. Even if you *know* you are safe, your body may still respond to change, perceived threats and real threats as they occur. When your body senses a perceived danger, it will cause your sympathetic nervous system to trigger the fight or flight response. This process has historically promoted safety for birthing women. When there is a sudden spike in these stress hormones, the heart beats faster, breathing becomes more rapid and there is a redistribution of blood toward vital organs, including the heart, lungs and major muscle groups.[2] This redistribution means there is less blood flowing to non-essential organs, including the uterus. These physiological changes are what would slow or completely stop contractions so our ancient relatives could fight or flee and find safety during the labor process.

While we no longer live during a time when we need to be fearful of a bear or tiger pouncing on us while we are trying to give birth, our body still takes in information and responds to situations that we perceive as threats in our birth space. The "bear in the forest" may now have become the internal vaginal exam, bright lights or noise in the busy hospital corridor. It is important to understand this aspect of birth hormones so you and your birth partner can prepare for and reduce situations that may put the breaks on birth. If you notice your contractions are beginning to space out more or have become very mild, it is helpful to assess how you are feeling and if anything in your environment needs to change.

How do you keep stress hormone levels low? Think of things that your body may *view* as potentially disruptive or unsettling and work out how you can reduce them. A change of scene, such as moving from home to the hospital can create anxiety for a laboring person. The car journey tends to be uncomfortable and the setting of a hospital is not very oxytocin-inducing. Bright lights, new smells, people rushing around, being asked questions during challenging contractions—all of these can cause an influx of stress hormones. Once you have identified a potentially stressful scenario, like this one, you can then work backwards to see how you could create a better sense of calm and comfort. See the tips below.

Our bodies produce more oxytocin when we feel safe, private and connected. During birth, one of the practical things your birth partner or doula can do is set the scene. Talk to them about what types of things would make *you* feel safe and cozy. This varies for everyone, but consider your five senses:

- What can you **see**? Most people prefer dim lighting, no overhead hospital lights unless necessary and maybe even add in some (fake) candles. Do you have affirmations, pictures or a special item you would like to look at as you labor? Something sentimental that may help. Some expecting parents create beautiful vision boards that can act as an oxytocin-boosting focal point. A vision board can be used at home or made to a portable size which can then be brought to a hospital or birth center. If you are having a cesarean, would you like clear drapes (if available) or the drapes to be lowered so you can see your baby emerge?
- What can you **hear**? Regular interruptions, the beeps of medical equipment, strangers talking in halls and idle chatter can mess with the flow of labor. Also be mindful that your senses might be heightened so even whispers may be annoying. You can use noise-cancelling headphones, play your own music, hypnobirthing tracks or guided meditations to help you block out any background noise. Do you want vocal encouragement and words of praise during labor or do you think you will prefer silence? Do not be afraid to tell people what you need in the moment and your needs may change as labor progresses.
- What can you **feel**? Have you prepared comfortable clothing to labor in? Wearing a hospital gown, if offered one, is optional. Do you

want a fan or cool face cloth if you become warm? Would you like to ensure you are covered for most of labor? Do you want people to ask before touching you? Bringing items from home like a pillow, blanket or sentimental item can be very soothing if you are giving birth in a hospital or birth center. I once had a client who held onto her grandmother's prayer beads during birth, which helped her feel connected to the women who had birthed before her.

- What **smells** are present in your birth space? Are you being overwhelmed by disinfectants in a hospital setting? Do you love the smell of essential oils, your partner's cologne or perfume? Put those in your birth bag! A room spray, scented candle, incense or essential oils diffuser may also be nice additions for a home birth. Much like your other senses, your sense of smell may be heightened during labor.
- Do not forget about the importance of **taste**! Our bodies create oxytocin when we eat and food energizes the body during labor. Despite what some hospitals may suggest, withholding food from a laboring person is not backed by science. Consider packing snacks in your labor bag or having easy-to-eat food at home if that is where you choose to birth. Research has shown that people tend to naturally eat less as labor progresses, so it would be completely normal to experience more hunger during earlier stages of labor.

My hope for all birthing people is that you will have a support person (or two!) who will take care of literally *everything else* so you can focus solely on your labor and getting through each contraction, one at a time. As labor progresses, most people will begin to turn inward and find a rhythm that helps get through each contraction. This shift can often be spotted when a mother begins to focus less on what is happening around her.

Many birth partners want to help during all stages of labor but may not know *how*. They may also feel like there is a lot of responsibility on their shoulders, which can feel overwhelming or scary. These feelings are normal, however, let's not forget that birth partners have an amazing opportunity to be involved in one of life's most memorable events. All of the information they need to provide support with confidence can be learned through prenatal education, books and/or online resources. Many of the oxytocin-promoting suggestions above overlap with other elements of physical, emotional and practical support that a birth partner can provide in any setting.

PHYSICAL SUPPORT

This may be provided throughout all of the labor process. This element of care ensures you are comfortable and aims to reduce the intensity of labor. During each stage of labor birth partners can utilize comfort measures, including: massage, acupressure and applying counterpressure. These hands-on techniques promote oxytocin release and can be used during or between contractions, as preferred. Learning these comfort measures during pregnancy allows time for practice, figuring out which methods appeal most to you and makes them easier for your birth partner to recall on the day. Some birth partners create small pocket guides or even use flashcards that they can reference once labor begins. You can learn these comfort measures by accessing online resources (especially videos), books and childbirth education. If you hire a doula, they will know all of these techniques inside and out so they can perform them themselves or provide guidance on when and how your birth partner can use them to your advantage.

Other types of physical support include helping you change positions while laboring or during the pushing phase, providing physical comfort (holding a hand, giving a hug) and helping you get in or out of a birth pool. If you are utilizing any equipment, such as a birth ball, peanut ball, labor wrap (sometimes called a Rebozo) or birthing stool, your birth partner can help with placement and getting these items for you when needed.

EMOTIONAL SUPPORT

This type of support helps birthing people feel safe, cared for and can create a sense of pride and empowerment following birth. You are more likely to reflect positively on your birth when your birth partner looks out for your emotional health. Many birthing people feel a sense of reassurance when they have the continuous presence of a support person. Emotional support may also include elements of praise, encouragement and showing a caring attitude. If labor becomes challenging, emotional support may involve reminding you of your strength, providing words of encouragement, asking what you need *right now,* assisting with focus (breathing in sync, or counting aloud during contractions) and actively working to ensure all of your choices during the labor process are respected. You deserve to know that your birth partner is by your side and on your side, ready to assist you and ensure your needs are met.

PRACTICAL SUPPORT

When your birth partner takes care of the practical aspects of birth, you will have more time and energy to focus on the labor process. While this aspect of support may not seem that important, the reality is people are better able to relax and let go when they know the finer details of their experience are being handled appropriately. The practicalities of birth differ depending on everyone's unique circumstance but may include the following: ensuring everything is packed for the hospital, timing contractions, knowing where all labor-support items are, inflating and filling a birth pool, ensuring childcare is arranged, calling a midwife or doula, offering food and drink, organizing music or hypnobirthing tracks and setting the scene for birth with any desired items.

Doing all of these practical things can create a sense of relief and keep oxytocin levels high because you will trust everything has already been taken care of. Ensure that you and your birth partner have a conversation about when you would like some of these practical things done—when you would like them to ring the hospital or midwife, when you want older siblings collected or brought elsewhere, etc.

OTHER TOPICS TO CONSIDER

How would you like your birth partner to communicate with caregivers if you are unable to or choose not to, so you can remain "in the zone" of oxytocin? Would you like them to take the conversation outside the room, or speak quietly so you can overhear?

How can they help you relax if you become anxious or have a "wobble" during labor? Would you like your birth partner to breathe in-sync with you? Is there a playlist they can put on? Are there affirmations you would like them to say? Would a hand on your shoulder help you feel grounded and safe? You may not know what will help until the day labor begins, and that is okay. Discussing what you think you might want is a good place to start, though.

What are your actual preferences for birth? What is your "ideal" birth?

How do you feel about pain relief? Laboring in water? Eating and drinking? What are your biggest fears? Your birth partner should know your birth plan inside and out so they feel better able to ask important questions and advocate for what it is *you* want from your experience.

Having open communication with your birth partner is key. Labor flows so much better when you feel connected and in-tune with one another. Preparing for labor is something you can certainly do together during the weeks and months leading up to birth. Schedule in some time to go over your ideas and practice any techniques you might want to try, like counterpressure or massage. If your birth partner is not your intimate partner, this is still an important step even if you cannot practice techniques as regularly.

I have been at births where the mom and birth partner barely spoke. They communicated beautifully with body language and whispered phrases, "A bit higher. Right there. You're safe. Breathe with me," often guided by intuition. It is incredible to watch two people coming together and working together as they follow the rhythm of birth.

DOULA SUPPORT

Chances are that if you have dipped your toe into the world of birth, you have come across the idea of hiring a doula. Doula support is definitely becoming more common, although many people still do not understand what a doula does or how they *really* help parents prepare for a positive experience. There are several different types of doulas, the most popular being birth and postpartum.

A birth doula is a trained professional who provides evidence-based information and education to expecting parents and supports them both emotionally and physically during labor. They usually meet with parents during pregnancy to help them prepare for birth, attend the birth wherever it takes place (hospital, home or birth center) and meet at least once following birth to check in with the new parents. A doula literally puts their life on hold so they can support parents whenever labor starts. Every doula is different in what they offer in terms of the number of prenatal visits and many have a range of package options. Others have service add-ons like lactation support, hypnobirthing, placenta encapsulation and more depending on their additional areas of expertise. Some doulas also offer virtual support throughout pregnancy and birth with all aspects of care being conducted via video chat, phone, text and email.

WHAT DOES THIS SUPPORT LOOK LIKE?

- **Education:** A doula will help you learn about all of your options for pregnancy and birth. They are experienced in supporting families from many different backgrounds and during all types of birth. Part of the education they offer may include common challenges you may face and how to avoid them or work through them. Both you and your birth partner will learn *practical tools* to help you manage the intensity of labor and how to *ensure your voice is heard* during the process.

- **Physical Support:** The vast majority of people prefer some form of physical support during labor. This may come in the form of counterpressure, massage, helping you change position, getting food or water and so much more! Doulas also provide reassurance to partners, may offer suggestions on how they can support you in the moment and boost their confidence in supporting you. Even if a doula is not actively "doing anything," the physical presence of someone you know and trust in the room can create a level of calm and keep stress levels down.

- **Emotional Support:** Birth is a journey. A birthing person and their partner may experience highs, lows and exhaustion. Your doula is always by your side, cheering you on, boosting your confidence and reminding you of the absolute powerhouse you are! They know techniques to help you feel safe, enhance your birth hormones and help you focus on birthing your baby, no matter what path your labor may take. They support your decisions and *have full faith in your ability to birth.*

DO YOU NEED A DOULA?

Many people have a supportive partner, family member or friend who is available and willing to support them on the day. They can absolutely be an invaluable support to you. However, doulas truly are experienced guides on the entire birth process. They understand the physiology of birth and know what resources and techniques may be the most helpful and when. A doula does not *replace* the role of your partner or other birth support, they are experts at *enhancing* their ability to care for you so you have a cohesive team of support.

A doula does not replace the advice of a medical professional, but they do guide you along the decision-making process to ensure you are at the center of your care. They are a constant support, especially in a busy hospital setting and during the normal hustle and bustle of birth. Many parents in a hospital setting assume a labor and delivery nurse will be taking on a primarily support role, however, research does not support this. Labor and delivery nurses often have to spread their time across many coexisting tasks: looking after more than one laboring person, adjusting and monitoring equipment, keeping records, administering medication, changing shifts and more.

One study showed labor and delivery nurses spend as little as 6% of their time providing direct labor support.[3] This is something to consider if you are planning to birth in a hospital. If you are deciding between hospitals, one question you may like to ask is if a midwife or nurse will be specifically assigned to you or if their shift will be spent looking after other people as well. While a labor and delivery nurse or midwife may have limited time with you, a doula is a constant source of support for both you and your birth partner.

WHAT THE RESEARCH SAYS

There are many research findings that show there are benefits to both parents and babies when birth doula support is utilized. A 2017 Cochrane Review showed:

- 39% decrease in cesarean risk

- 15% increase in likelihood of spontaneous vaginal birth
- 10% decrease in medication for pain relief
- Decreased length of labor, averaging at 41 minutes
- 38% decrease in the baby's risk of a low five-minute Apgar score
- 31% decreased risk of being dissatisfied with one's birth experience
- 54% reduction in synthetic oxytocin (Pitocin or syntocinon) use to speed up or start labor [1]

Doula support is also associated with lower pain levels during labor and a reduction in anxiety levels for first-time moms.[4] The American College of Obstetricians and Gynecologists (ACOG) has clinical guidelines on the *Safe Prevention of the Primary Cesarean Delivery* which was created to provide guidance on how to reduce the cesarean rate for first-time moms and thus address the concerning cesarean rate which continues to climb in the United States. Within this document, the ACOG states, "Published data indicate that one of the most effective tools to improve labor and delivery outcomes is the continuous presence of support personnel, such as a doula."[5]

COST AND HOW TO FIND ONE

The cost of doula support often depends on your location and the experience of the doula you are seeking. Their price includes not only their time with you in-person but covers the cost of typical business expenses that any practitioner would have: business registration, insurance, transportation costs, further training, maintaining certification, being on call and more. Most doulas are on call for your birth for four to five weeks *minimum*, meaning they are available to attend your labor at a moment's notice. When a doula is on call for you also keep in mind that *someone is often on call for them,* especially if they have children and require childcare. The average cost of a doula is often somewhere between $800-1500, depending on the number of visits and any extras. This may be fully or partially covered by some insurance policies. There are also doulas who offer sliding fee scales and large doula organizations may also offer a range of assistance programs.

A good internet search or referral from a friend or family member can often help you find a doula. Many doula training organizations also have directories you can search by location. I recommend interviewing more than one doula before hiring anyone since they will be supporting you during a very personal and vulnerable time. You are the only person who knows whether having a doula feels like the right option for you. There are so many birth professionals ready to support you as you journey to meet your baby.

The closer I get to my baby's estimated birth date, the more confident I feel.

Giving birth, no matter what path your labor may take, is one of the most powerful and amazing things you will ever experience. Meeting your precious baby for the first time will bring on life's largest surge of oxytocin and a moment you will never forget. Ask any person who has given birth about what their birth experience was like and I can guarantee you they will remember the "big moments," but they will also remember some of the most minute details—whether it was a sound, smell or something that was said to them lovingly. As you enter the early days with your baby, your heart will continue to expand as the love for your child grows through the difficulties, overwhelm and beautiful memories you create together. I am so excited for you and the journey that lies ahead!

I hope you now feel more informed, prepared and confident about all aspects of birth and the amazing capacity your body has to see you through. Your body was built for this! Learning to appreciate your body and all of the changes that occur throughout pregnancy may take time. I hope you know that no matter how your body changes, those changes are significant and part of your story. No person's story or path to birth is exactly the same.

Please revisit Part One of this book to access all of the hints, tips and tools that will help you navigate becoming a parent. I know life is busy and if you need to step away from these materials for a while, you can always come back to them. I hope you take away from this book that you now have full ownership over all of the decisions relating to your body, your baby and your birth. Only you know what feels right for you at any given moment. You now have the tools to advocate for yourself clearly and with confidence, whether that is during pregnancy or the labor process.

I urge you to continue preparing yourself for birth, no matter what that looks like for you. Here are some suggestions:

- Sign up for size-friendly childbirth education
- Assess your local provider options
- Sign up for a hypnobirthing class online or in-person
- Hire a size-friendly doula
- Find more positive birth resources: books, affirmation cards or tracks, birth stories and videos
- Engage in movement that makes you feel good: yoga, pilates, walking, water aerobics and more

You will find a significant list of resources at the back of this book to help you get started. Do not forget to engage with communities and other expecting parents who are navigating pregnancy at the same time. Do be mindful about the discussions taking place within those groups and give yourself permission to step away if the language or themes are either fatphobic or depicting birth in very negative ways. It is okay to set boundaries and continue surrounding yourself with depictions of birth that are more aligned with your vision. The more you immerse yourself within these environments and access positive resources, the more confident you will become and you will feel more supported as you get closer to giving birth.

Read on for a rich collection of birth stories submitted by plus size parents from all over the world. There is a large variety of experiences, types of birth and of course everyone who shared their story has come from a different background. These new parents had positive births with healthy outcomes and that is a possibility for you, too. I hope you enjoy them!

Head over to www.fatandpregnant.com/shop and enter code **FATBIRTHBOOK** to get your free body positive affirmations MP3 that you can listen to throughout pregnancy whenever you need a reminder of just how amazing your body is.

Content Warnings:
Some of the birth stories contained within Part Two mention difficult situations which some may find triggering. Please take note of the content warnings at the start of each story. They may include: weight stigma within medical settings, mention of exact weight, obstetric violence, pregnancy loss and more.

PART TWO:

BIRTH STORIES

FAT BIRTH

Sarah, United States

The path to pregnancy was filled with a lot of anxiety for my husband and me. This was partly because of my weight and also because of my husband's previous experience with infertility during a prior marriage. After having my IUD removed and "trying" around my most fertile time, I ended up becoming pregnant the first month it was possible. I had no idea conception would be that easy, so we didn't realize I was pregnant until almost seven weeks.

I had an incredible pregnancy, despite the fact I experienced exhaustion and nausea through the first trimester. It was challenging, but I was able to rest when needed. By the second trimester, I felt great and I hired a personal trainer who specialized in prenatal training. At the beginning of the pregnancy, I saw an obstetrician a couple of times as well. This doctor had a great reputation, and his office was very understanding when I requested that I not be told my weight at any appointments. I also requested that my weight not be discussed unless absolutely necessary for my medical care. When we discussed my birth preferences, I mentioned that I anticipated wanting to push in whatever position my body called for. He responded by saying that it makes it truly hard for him when women squat or are on hands and knees because he has to lie on the floor. I thought that was bullshit—you think lying on the floor is hard? Try pushing out a baby on your back! I immediately switched to a hospital-based midwifery practice, assuming that all aspects of my care would improve.

While the midwives were more supportive of mom-led birthing, I had some real issues with them related to my weight. Having to ask at every visit for a blind weigh-in always stressed me out and drove my blood pressure up. I found it is so stressful to be fat in any medical setting and they always wanted to take my blood pressure after being weighed. Things only got worse. At my twenty-week visit, a midwife told me my weight. It was right before my husband and I were leaving for our babymoon in Switzerland and Paris, and I was devastated. The midwife told me my weight gain had been "perfect," but hearing the number sent me into the spiral I was hoping to avoid with blind weigh-ins. Prior to that, I had felt extremely good in and about my body. Being told my weight despite requesting a blind weigh-in felt so violating and disrespectful.

At that same prenatal visit, we had our twenty-week anatomy scan. Everything looked perfect, but the doctor asked us to schedule a thirty-week scan on our way out. We didn't understand why, but the office was about to close so we scheduled it and went home to pack for our vacation. I put the whole bad experience out of my mind. On the day we were flying home from Paris, the detailed report of my ultrasound was posted on my online health account. I saw that the thirty-week scan was indicated *solely* based on my body mass index. I knew BMI to be an extremely flawed measure, intended for population-wide analysis of food availability and not individual health. I was livid. I also knew that later ultrasounds, which are incredibly inaccurate, often resulted in doctors becoming concerned about "large babies." My husband and I dove into the research papers during our layover in New York. It was absolutely clear to us that we would not be consenting to an unnecessary, and, likely, inaccurate second ultrasound based solely on my BMI.

At my next appointment, I discussed my concerns with the midwife—the fact that I felt violated when my express wish to not be told my weight was ignored for no reason and the fact that I was not told the reason for the recommended thirty-week scan. Ultimately, the midwife responsible apologized half-heartedly. We decided to continue care with them but also explore other options. We met with another obstetrician who seemed like an even worse fit, after telling me that all moms get an epidural!

In January we started thinking about backup plans for our late April due date. By March, we had hired a "backup" home-birth midwife. For us, the data suggested that a certified nurse-doula (CNM) was the safest option, given that this was my first birth experience. The rates of adverse outcomes with a CNM attending a home birth are actually very similar to the rates in most hospitals. We ended up falling totally in love with our midwife, Naomi, and instead of retaining her service as a backup plan, she became our primary care provider.

I definitely had to go through a process of fear and worry about being at home for birth. Without the "safety net" of an anesthesiologist around the corner, I knew I was diving into something huge. I had been preparing for the lowest-intervention birth that would be safely possible, so it was not that big of a change. I was super excited to plan on being at home where I knew I would feel much safer and less stressed than in a medical setting. My blood pressure goes up just walking into a doctor's office, a place where I have been shamed and belittled for my body's shape and size since I was an early teen. Having a home birth with a supportive team was the best and safest option for me and my baby.

I was losing my mind and so ready for labor to begin as my due date passed on Monday, April 27th. I couldn't understand how labor could just spontaneously begin and was dealing with a huge amount of anxiety that it would not. We had planned to medically induce labor at forty-one weeks if it did not start on its own. After reviewing some statistics, I knew that if labor had not begun naturally by forty weeks, I had about a 50 percent chance of it starting before forty-one weeks. I really did not want to be induced at the hospital and I cried every night.

The Saturday before my due date, I thought my waters broke. I'd had some cramping early that morning, so when I felt some fluid that was definitely not pee, I thought it could be my waters. I was excited that we might be having the baby but I also knew it was not ideal for my membranes to rupture before contractions started. We had our midwife come and drop off the amniotic fluid test because our birth kit had of course been missing that one item. It turned out not to be amniotic fluid—a relief, but it meant we were back to the waiting game. On Tuesday, I had an acupuncture appointment to help bring on labor, as well as a chiropractic adjustment. I cried a lot more that evening in the shower and spoke out loud to my baby. I told him I was sorry I had been putting so much pressure on him and that I trusted him to come when he was ready. I told him how scared I was of going to the hospital and how much I wanted to gently welcome him to the world in a peaceful environment.

On Wednesday morning I woke up at 4:30 a.m. feeling some cramping and mild practice contractions. I used the bathroom and went back to bed to try to sleep. I was trying very hard not to get my hopes up as I'd had some middle of the night cramping earlier in the week that disappeared by morning. I dozed on and off until around 7 a.m. When I got up, I still felt crampy. I texted my husband, Aaron, and we both agreed it was a good sign but that it could also be nothing. I decided to stay busy and watered the plants and started some laundry. At 9 a.m., I texted our birth team that I thought some "early action" may be happening. I said I didn't want to use the word "contraction" yet. I continued my housework and planned a walk with my mom. At 10 a.m., I texted our midwife team again that contractions were lasting thirty to forty-five seconds at ten minutes apart. I went for a walk with my mom shortly after and the contractions became way more intense. I had to stop three times during our two block circle to lean on a street sign.

When we got home, I called Aaron in from his "work from home" office in the garage studio. I then texted the birth team to see if I should keep my acupuncture appointment at noon and updated them that contractions were closer to five minutes apart. By the time the acupuncturist arrived late at 12:30 p.m., I needed to move through every wave to cope with the intensity. My doula and midwife arrived at the same time as the acupuncturist. It was hard to lie still with the needles in for thirty minutes. Aaron sat with me through the acupuncture on our bed and told me it was okay if I needed the needles out sooner to move. I wanted to stick it out, though, knowing that acupuncture can help progression of labor and with pain management.

After we finally finished with that, the midwife did an internal exam and we found out I was completely effaced and 3-4 cm dilated! I was thrilled as I felt like "labor" had really gotten started around noon. They asked me how I felt about the dilation, meaning how far along I was, and what story I was telling myself. I was just happy labor was underway and the sensations definitely were not Braxton Hicks.

The midwife said she was going to leave for a while and come back. By this point contractions were very intense and lasting a minute. Aaron and our doula, Laura, followed my lead. I had to move through each one and was vocalizing as well. The contractions felt like the kind of horrible menstrual cramps that make you feel like you have to make a bowel movement, just stronger as time went on. I felt them in my thighs and stomach, where I usually experienced menstrual cramps.

Since we were hanging out on and around the toilet, Laura suggested I try sitting on it backwards for more support. There wasn't room for this in the master bathroom so we moved to the powder room. Laura asked if music sounded good, and I said yes. Aaron put on one of my birth playlists. He chose the "birth party" list—*Oh my god, what is he thinking that he thought this might be the right mood?* He switched it to my Jewish holy music playlist and we ended up with that on repeat until Sam was born.

I was not very interested in physical touch, which Aaron and Laura tried a bit of while we were in the powder room. The key thing for me was being ready and bracing myself as I felt the contraction begin. This was a mental thing as well as being in a stable physical position where I could move through the intensity. I breathed intentionally through them and moaned a lot, trying to stay in a low register.

At some point Laura encouraged us to try another position and we moved to the shower. Being in the shower felt great, but I still felt like I had to be on my hands and knees. I came out and we tried some positions in the bedroom. Lying down in the bed was clearly a complete non-starter for me, but I did lean over the ball for a while. Contractions were fast and sometimes seemed to come in a set of two or three with barely a break to catch my breath. My music, birth art and mantras all helped and I felt so relieved that I would not have to be induced at the hospital. I was proud to be moving through the flow of labor and just focusing on each moment as it came.

Laura was nervous that my knees would get sore and that I would get exhausted supporting myself on hands and knees for so long. I was feeling pretty okay strength-wise, but her concern did make me start to worry a bit about whether I would tire using the only coping mechanism that worked for me. I got into the shower for the second time to try a different position and give myself a break from hands and knees. Laura was not in the bathroom with me and Aaron left for a bit. I felt abandoned and alone. When Aaron came back less than five minutes later, I told him I could not be alone. I needed him or Laura by my side all the time.

Laura asked what I wanted to do next—bath or try the bed again. Clearly bath. They filled the tub and I did get relief through one, or maybe two contractions after getting in the water. Laura told me the midwife was on her way and asked me if she could leave and take a work call out in the garage studio. I remember saying, "Can I say no?" and she remembers me just saying, "NO."

The only time I questioned whether I would be able to birth my baby at home was when I was in the bath. *If I'm still only 4-5 cm when the midwife checks me again,* I thought, *I'm going to need to get an epidural so I can get some rest.* At the same time, I could not imagine getting in the car to go to the hospital. I put that scenario out of my mind as an unsolvable problem at that point.

Immediately after, I had an insane contraction that made me get up and try to get on my hands and knees again. I was looking down into the bathwater and saw something dark. "What's that?" I asked.

My doula said, "I think your water just broke."

There was some meconium in the amniotic fluid, so we all agreed I needed to get out of the bath. Once my waters had released, I felt like I needed to push during contractions. I decided to go back into the shower to rinse off some of the meconium. Don't push yet, you may not be fully dilated, I thought to myself. I was nervous about pushing before my body was ready and getting a swollen cervix.

It felt like forever before the midwife arrived, and she was definitely (calmly) rushing to get set up once she saw the shape I was in. During a contraction, I said I felt like I needed to push, and she told me I did not need to fight my body. She brought a super-calm energy, and when she checked me I was almost 10 cm! She said I had a tiny rim in the front of the cervix that needed to open, probably because I had been bent over on hands and knees basically the entire labor. She told me to do a few contractions standing up. While I was doing that, her assistant arrived, also scrambling to get into the room and her hands washed. She said I could push, but I asked her to check my cervix again to make sure. In my head, for some reason, I was chanting, "No swollen cervix."

I pushed leaning over the side of our bed. It felt great to really push. I pushed for about thirty minutes and then his head came out. I definitely felt the burning sensation, but compared to the contractions, it was bearable. My midwife was stretching me with warm oil and compresses—something I had hoped for and envisioned. Her assistant checked Sam's heart rate, which sounded perfect, and was a huge relief. I remember it felt like a long time between when his head was out and my next contraction/urge to push. I didn't feel I could push between and my birth team just told me to listen to my body. I asked if he was okay and they said he was fine. I was relieved when he was born after the next push!

When he cried there was not an immediate rush of emotion other than pure relief. I wanted to make sure he was okay and get him to latch as soon as he was ready. I also kept track of needing to birth the placenta, which happened on its own during a contraction fifteen minutes later.

Immediately after was a time out of time. I cannot really remember any thoughts—just joy and the closeness to God that I had hoped to feel as I snuggled with Aaron and Sam. My parents came to meet their first grandbaby shortly after. There was plenty of activity but I felt cocooned, respected and safe. Eventually the midwife put in a couple of stitches. She said they were optional but I didn't want to take any chances.

Latching was difficult and there was some stress about that, but Sam did manage to eat a bit. We were so thrilled we'd had a quick, low-intervention labor and a healthy newborn baby at home!

Tammy Mondeci, United States:

I discovered I was pregnant when I least expected it. After a decade of irregular cycles and a diagnosis of polycystic ovarian syndrome, I wasn't sure if having a biological child would ever be in my future. Following a relationship breakdown, I had started to pray very hard for God to help me conceive. I wanted to experience the unconditional love felt between a mother and child. I never lost hope that I would get pregnant.

At forty-two years old and after two years without having a period, my cycle returned in August 2017. It came again in October, so I assumed I would get another in December. When my period still hadn't arrived in January, I started thinking I might be pregnant. I went and got a test after work and decided to take it at home. My friend was living with me at the time and I didn't tell her I was taking it. It immediately showed a solid, positive line, and I told my friend the news through my tears. I called my mom and when I told her how quick the test turned positive, she said I might be further along than I thought. I called my gynecologist's office next and they could not get me in for six weeks, which I was not happy with. I contacted a free clinic and got in to see them within a few days. I took another pregnancy test there and I was so nervous—*what if it comes back negative?*

It came back positive again and I started crying in the office. I had in the back of my mind—*this may not be true.* The clinic scheduled me for an ultrasound a week later and the tech told me I was eleven weeks and six days pregnant! As soon as I saw my baby on the screen, she was jumping around and so big already. I never had any early pregnancy symptoms, other than gagging once while I brushed my teeth.

I had no complications during the rest of my pregnancy, although people made comments about my pregnancy and body. Some people at work told me I didn't look pregnant, as if that was a compliment, and others told me I would end up with gestational diabetes. When I told those coworkers I had taken the gestational diabetes test and it was negative, they seemed surprised—they clearly assumed all people who are plus size will have it. Sometimes they commented on my food choices and said things like, "Should you be eating that?" They finally stopped after I told them to stop being the food police.

The only negative symptom I experienced during my pregnancy was carpal tunnel syndrome. I would wake up at night with numb hands or have sharp pains in my wrists, especially if I tried to pick something up. It started around thirty-seven weeks and happened mostly when I was asleep. My baby was also breech for most of my pregnancy, which had me concerned about being scheduled for a cesarean. Thankfully, she had turned by my last ultrasound scan so I could try for a vaginal birth.

My mom, two sisters and niece came to Texas on July 21st, less than a week before my induction. My doctor did offer me a cesarean, which I declined. I went in on the 25th and arrived at the hospital at 7 p.m. I was a bit nervous about labor and I was trying not to get too stressed about it. Cervidil was inserted at 9 p.m. and I started feeling contractions by 10 p.m. They didn't feel how I thought they would—they weren't coming and going but were more constant. It was not unbearable, but the contractions were very uncomfortable. The longer they went on the more intense they became. I had to really focus on my breathing so I wasn't getting much time to sleep.

My mom and sister, Christina, were in the room with me and I had a nurse with me the entire time. The nurse was talking to me and helping me get my mind off labor a bit, which was helpful. During this time I was alternating between the bed, walking around my room and sitting on the birth ball. I couldn't leave the room because I was using the wireless fetal monitor. It was great to talk with my mom and Christina, who kept the mood up and got me laughing.

The Cervidil was removed the following morning at 9 a.m. and the doctor did an internal exam. I was 1 cm dilated and seventy-five percent effaced. I could hardly believe it. I thought for sure my cervix would be more dilated after the Cervidil had been in for twelve hours. Knowing what I know now, I honestly don't think my body and baby were ready for labor to begin. I think that's why it took so long for my body to begin dilating.

My doctor asked me about the epidural and reminded me that I could get it at any point if I wanted. I told her I would think about it and was started on Pitocin at noon. I was afraid to be receiving it, as I had heard some negative stories about its use and how it could make labor more intense. Once I started on it, however, I enjoyed the change because the Pitocin eased the constant feeling of discomfort. Instead of the constant intensity with the Cervidil, Pitocin created much more of a pattern so I was able to get breaks between the contractions. The nurses were great at bringing me ice pops, gelatin and ice water to keep my energy levels up during this time.

At 2:30 p.m. I was still 1 cm dilated and again, the doctor told me I could opt for an epidural if I wanted to. I found the internal exams very painful and was told having the epidural would help ease the pain of them, so I decided to go for it. My waters were broken too, and the anesthesiologist arrived to perform my epidural at 3:30 p.m. The nurse was with me and I was surprised at how fast and easy it was to insert the epidural. I was so happy I got it. I was able to relax, sleep and the nurses helped move me from side to side with a cushion between my legs. They helped me switch sides every hour and I think being able to relax my body more helped things progress.

It was about 1:15 a.m. when I started to feel pressure on my bladder and the nurse did another internal exam. I was 7 cm dilated and ninety percent effaced. I was so happy I had dilated that far over the course of the night. I started to feel more and more pressure and at my next internal exam, I was 8 cm dilated. My doctor came to the room at 3 a.m. and I was still feeling the pressure on my bladder, versus my bowels like everyone describes. I was now 9 cm dilated and the nurses turned down the epidural so I would have a return in sensation and be better able to push. With the epidural turned down, I was certainly able to feel more and the urge to push began. I was fully dilated and ready to push at 3:30 a.m., when I was instructed to use my abdominal muscles for more effective pushing.

It felt like I was pushing for a long time compared to other family members whose births I had been at, but in reality, I was only pushing for about thirty minutes. I pushed twelve times before my daughter's head came out. It was incredibly hard not to continue pushing when I felt the "ring of fire" of her crowning.

When my daughter first arrived, I was stunned and almost felt like I was in shock for a moment. Considering how long my labor was, things seemed to move very quickly once she was born. I told the hospital staff that I wanted to have immediate skin to skin and delayed cord clamping, however, I did not have her on my chest as long as I wanted initially. They gave Amayah to me for a short time and then had to take her to the side to help her breathe. They suctioned her once and brought her to me but had to bring her to the warmer a second time for more suctioning. My sister cut the umbilical cord, Amayah was returned to me, and I started breastfeeding shortly after.

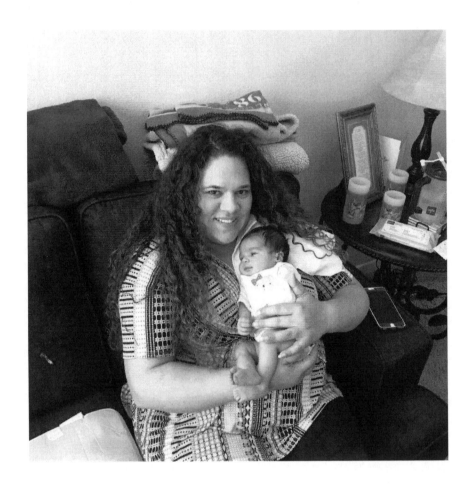

Anonymous:

*** Content warning for weight stigma within a medical setting and mention of weight loss.*

My pregnancy journey was an arduous and painful one. It started with a frustrating six-year period of unexplained infertility. I was plus size during my infertility struggles, but no one made an issue about it—except my husband. He really believed that I couldn't conceive because I was "too big." I explained countless times that bigger women conceive just as well as straight size people.

My husband brought my weight up with the consultant during one of our appointments and she politely said that losing weight would indeed increase my chances of conceiving. She never mentioned it again. Throughout all of our infertility tests, procedures and appointments during those six years, not one medic pulled me up on my weight.

When I finally fell pregnant at the age of thirty-four, we were beyond shocked. I did four tests just to be sure! We found out just before Christmas so it took a while before I was able to see my general practitioner. She was very happy for us, as she knew about our struggle to conceive.

Our elation lasted until I was diagnosed with both high blood pressure and gestational diabetes. Again, no one blamed my weight on those issues nor resorted to scaremongering—until I went for a scan mid-pregnancy.

The ultrasound technician at my appointment was visibly annoyed that I was plus size and said it was difficult for her to see the baby because there was, "So much fat to get through." I explained that I had actually lost weight because of gestational diabetes but she said it did not make a difference. "You would have to lose a ton of weight for me to be able to see your baby properly." Disheartened and ashamed, I soldiered on.

The gestational diabetes left me tired and hungry. I was testing five times a day and injecting myself with insulin. I survived on cheese, nuts, egg mayo and Ryvitas. I had serious carb envy and disliked my husband being able to eat anything he wanted.

The pregnancy took its toll on me mentally and physically but I was still so grateful and excited about the person growing in my belly—a belly I had hated and been embarrassed about for most of my life. I saw my consultants every week on account of the gestational diabetes. They were all happy with the baby's growth and size. I had always wanted a cesarean but they did not think it was necessary.

My final pregnancy scan was with the same fat shaming ultrasound technician. I was still hopeful for a cesarean but she shot that down very quickly. She said that it was a bad idea because I risked heavy bleeding, it would be hard for the doctors to operate because of the size of my belly, I could break the bed in theater and worst of all—I could lose the baby. She said all this whilst doing my final scan.

I asked my consultant about everything and he was shocked. He downplayed everything she had said and did not take it seriously. I was annoyed that she had filled my head with negative, catastrophic thoughts just before the birth of my child. After we spoke to the consultant, we decided to make a complaint to the head midwife.

The head midwife called in the ultrasound tech who had performed my scan into a little room. My husband and I sat opposite the two of them like we were in a school principal's office. The head midwife explained that the ultrasound technician was a midwife too and a very experienced one who was only trying to help. The ultrasound technician said that she cared about my baby's wellbeing and that she has no problem with using the word "fat." That word was used a lot that day.

After hearing both sides, the head midwife sided with the ultrasound technician and said that I was just stressed and anxious because I was a first-time mum. She made me feel small about not knowing that the technician was a midwife too, and I apologized—although I'm still not sure why. The head midwife did say that cesareans do carry more risks and that heavy bleeding could happen to anyone. She said that she would ask the labor ward about the bed weight limit. She called them from her desk in the clinic and told us, in front of all the other pregnant women, that the limit was around 200 kg.

With that humiliation still playing heavily on my mind, my waters broke just a few days before my scheduled induction. I spent a whole night and day in the labor ward, strapped to a bed without food or sleep while they monitored my baby. Everything was fine and I was on track for a vaginal birth but with the gestational diabetes and lack of food and sleep, I knew I would not be able to go down that route. I asked the midwife to talk to the consultants about a cesarean and they relented.

I was prepped immediately and rushed to the operating room. It was all over so quickly. I remember crying when I heard my baby's cry, then eventually being wheeled to the postnatal ward.

None of the things the ultrasound technician said came true. It was a smooth and straightforward cesarean. My baby was perfectly fine and I did not have heavy bleeding. No one weighed me to check whether I would break the bed or operating table. My daughter was born small at 6 lbs 13 oz and never grew into the "giant baby" that was previously predicted.

Apart from that one ultrasound technician, every other medic during my pregnancy was polite, professional and positive. They had the emotional intelligence to appreciate my difficult conception and pregnancy journey. Many of them seemed genuinely happy for me when they came to see the baby and me in the postnatal ward.

Mary Guidone, United States:

*** Content warning for mention of weight loss,
disordered eating and exercise.*

I am a firstborn, and as a child, I very distinctly recall my siblings and I hearing the story of my mother's complicated first birth experience. She had heard over and over from her own mother how excruciatingly painful labor was—to the point where it completely terrified her. When my mother's labor with me began, her inability to relax and trust her own body contributed to nearly two days of no progress. As a result, she was brought in for a cesarean birth. This was followed by three successful vaginal births of my two sisters and my brother, but the story that bore frequent repeating was always mine. The trauma! The fear! It made for great, dramatic storytelling.

Even as a young child, I felt awful for my mother retelling it. I felt so sad for her experience—not the cesarean itself, but the fear put in her by my grandmother. My mother's story was less of a cautionary tale about medical intervention and more about how birth has been talked about and related to between generations. I am incredibly grateful that she didn't put the same fear into my siblings and me, and also that when it was my turn, my mother acted as my doula and birthing coach. Her support helped me achieve my ideal birthing experience.

My own birth story begins awhile before my actual pregnancy. In 2010, I was living in Chicago, Illinois USA. I had just finished graduate school and had been offered a one-year, full-time contract to teach at the college from which I had just graduated. It felt like absolutely everything was finally going right after such a stressful period being a student—except for one thing. I had gained a lot of weight during college and graduate school, and decided that enough was enough—I was going to change things! I developed a lot of disordered eating and exercise-related habits. Praise and congratulations from family, friends and co-workers kept me focused on these patterns of restriction.

One year later, almost exactly to the day, I was down 150 lbs. A few weeks later, I was offered a job in California and I moved there by the end of the summer. All these huge transitions were going on in my life and all I could think about was the scale, the numbers, the obsession. I maintained that weight for about a year through compulsive exercise, laxatives and other purging methods. I should have been happy, this is the body I want, right?—but I had never been more miserable or self-conscious in my life!

I returned to Chicago in the summer of 2012. Following an apartment mishap, I found myself living with the boyfriend I had dated before moving to the West Coast and had been seeing remotely. It was, unsurprisingly, a terrible idea. I needed to leave the situation but as I actively searched for apartments, I got a surprise.

After two years of such heavy regulation, measurement and obsession, I knew right away something was happening in my body. I was training for the Chicago Marathon and kept hitting a wall when I tried to run more than a few miles. I felt sore and tired in a way I had never felt before. After a late period, I got a pregnancy test from the drugstore down the block—and there it was.

Chicago was an incredible place to be an expectant mother. It is such a wonderful city with so many options, so much information and resources at your fingertips. I looked into the university where I had gone to graduate school, which I knew not only had a hospital and health system, but also a midwifery program. It was perfect—appointments and services from the midwives and delivery in their birth center within the hospital. An assisting doctor would be nearby if needed, but otherwise, I would be able to have the most natural experience possible.

I had my first appointment with a midwife around seven weeks and again a month later. In those few weeks I had gained nearly twenty pounds. I told myself I would be able to keep myself "under control," but all I knew was disorder. The restriction I had lived with before was not working anymore. I was so hungry, although most things smelled awful to me. I lived off crackers and hummus for days at a time. I tried running, but I would only get to a quarter-mile before becoming nauseated and sick. All the comfort of my routines was now gone and the smaller body I struggled to feel comfortable in was now becoming uncomfortable in a whole new way.

The midwife from my second appointment was condescending, basing my entire appointment on my weight rather than my bloodwork and test results. After a lifetime of avoiding doctors due to size anxiety, I remained quiet, feeling unable to assert myself. She told me foods to avoid, assuming I consumed high amounts of sugar and said my baby needed "real food."

I was doubly stunned when she handed me a sheet off her prescription pad where she simply wrote "Exercise!" At this stage I was struggling with meals and every time I needed to step on a scale. The Chicago Marathon came and went, and it was hard to keep calm and grieve that loss in a healthful way without her voice echoing in my mind.

I was much more vocal at my next appointment—I knew my body and its story, and I was doing the best that I could. This new midwife sat with me and listened for an hour as I told her about my eating disorder, weight loss, California and my relationship with my boyfriend. She made me feel heard, valued and best of all, treated me as an expert on my own situation. I made sure to always see her for future appointments.

I continued to steadily gain weight over the pregnancy. This is not undoing progress, I told myself. *This is my body when I actually eat.* I ate what I craved, as I wanted to make sure my baby was healthy and well-nourished. My blood work and all the tests were always in the normal, healthy ranges—no diabetes, no high blood pressure and an impressive resting heart rate due to the previous years of activity.

I was concerned about birth because of my size, but I tried to be as calm as possible—remembering the story of my mother. My midwife reassured me that my baby was fine and healthy. I was sent for extra ultrasounds for measurements and saw it only as a win. I got to see my baby much more before he was born than I would have done in a smaller body!

I was due at the end of April 2013. My mother flew in from Connecticut two days before my baby's estimated birth date and we started trying every old wives' tale in the book to start labor—long walks, spicy food, even castor oil. Nothing got my labor started and on May 5th, I was finally induced.

My body was bigger than when I got pregnant but I was also much more confident and assertive about myself and my baby. I had a birth plan prepared and said with certainty that I didn't want to receive an epidural. In our pre-birth Lamaze and hospital tour group, I had shared this to the gasps and disapproval of the other expecting mothers. Even the leader of the group laughed and shared that she had also wanted to avoid pain medicine during her births, but once labor had started, she changed her mind quickly. I didn't know if I would change my mind, but I wanted to at least be able to try. After three years of incredible body changes and transformations, I was struggling a lot with dysphoria. I had done so much to my body, not all good, that now I wanted to give myself one positive body experience. I wanted my body to be more than just the sum of weight added or subtracted, more than measurements or meals or miles. I wanted to feel *everything*.

I don't know how I would have done without my mother there. She coached me through labor, helping me breathe and reassuring me of my strength and competence. She helped me channel a confidence and tenacity of which I had never believed myself to be capable. She held my hand, rubbed my back, cooled my forehead and cheered for me well into the night. I will never forget—at one point I was having contractions so hard that I vomited. My mother, who has a notoriously weak stomach, did not flinch or bat an eye—she just held my hair and the trash can, believing in me through the sickness. I appreciated it as best I could at that moment. I only wish she had received the same strength and support from her own mother.

Almost twenty-four hours after we arrived at the hospital for my induction, my waters were broken and I was told it was time to begin pushing. Four good pushes, and there he was—a perfectly healthy, 7 lb 8 oz little chicken of a babe. The midwife placed him on my chest and I started sobbing, "My baby, my baby…" The whole thing was such a blur of amazement, marvel and wonder. *I did it. My body is large and impressive and capable of incredible things.*

I love that my mother's story of supporting me is much more joyful and proud than the story we heard of her first birth. She freely shares that my son was born face-up, and while he was still being birthed, he opened his eyes and looked at her. "He looked right at me!" she gushes. "He couldn't even wait to be fully born to start being curious!" My son, now seven years old, loves the story too, and I am so happy to have such a positive birth story to share with our family's next generation.

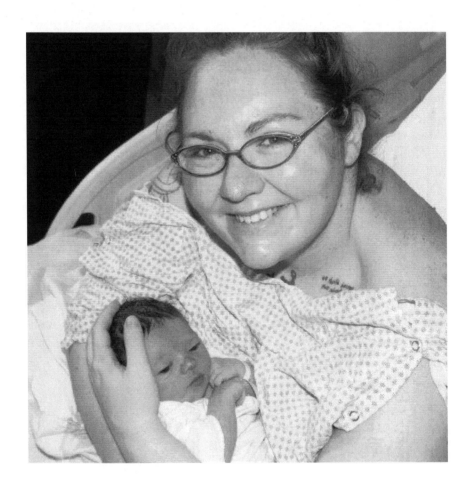

Liz Thomas, Wales:

I have always been on the plus size side of life—I have felt shame, judgment from society and much misunderstanding surrounding it over the years. Thankfully, my pregnancy and birth were not one of those times. I was fortunate to get everything I dreamed of—I manifested it. My dream came true in October 2018 when I birthed my little beauty into the world like the curvaceous goddess that I am.

I began pregnancy at the smallest size I had been in many years. A small size sixteen, I ended pregnancy at a large size eighteen. Although my partner and I had never tried to conceive in fourteen years of our relationship, we decided to go without contraception and see what happened. I conceived the first time without it!

As time passed, I adored being pregnant. I loved my belly and was proud of it for the first time in my life. I happily wore things that clung more and wore what I wanted without shame. I felt so in love with my body. I wanted a waterbirth but I had gained weight and was over the recommended BMI. I expected to face some adversity from my hospital trust—but I did not. I firmly expressed my plans and was met with respect and approval at all points.

My labor was all I could have wished for—early stages at home, latter stages in a midwife-led unit and eventually laboring in a pool. I was near-naked in front of strangers and I did not care. It was so empowering after years of hiding my body.

As my girl got closer to being born, I floated in and out of chatter and rest. I starfished in the pool as my body did the work, alongside conscious breath for my mind. My fatness did not matter—after all, I had just grown this human and I could birth it! It was spiritual, sacred and special. As my daughter emerged and for weeks after, all I could think about was how amazing my fat body was—strong and powerful. I felt like a goddess, having no pain relief, no intervention, no tearing and just looking into my partner's eyes for support. That moment I was way out of my body and realized, we are so capable—size says nothing about strength.

Samantha Ava Grace, England:

As we drew closer to my induction date on February 16th, it was becoming apparent that Zach would not be turning on his own. Despite my attempts to get him to flip, he remained in a breech position. I had a phone consultation with my doctor and she talked through the risks of attempting a vaginal breech birth—it did not look good. I reluctantly agreed that if a third ECV (external cephalic version) attempt did not work then I would have a planned cesarean. The ECV was booked for February 27th, when I was thirty-nine weeks pregnant.

We arrived in hospital on the Monday morning. I was so hopeful Zach would turn but deep down I think I knew that he would not. I knew either way that very soon my son would be born. We would either start an induction today if he turned or I would be going to theater for a cesarean if he did not.

We tried two more times to turn our baby boy head down, but he would not budge.

"You tried baby," my partner, Emmanuel, said to me as he held my hand.

We were checked in and given a private room where we would be staying until the cesarean. Then we waited. And waited and waited. It turns out that we would not be having our baby that day. The hospital informed us that they just could not fit us in. We decided to go for dinner and came back to the hospital later. The night was an odd one. We both knew what was coming but we were in limbo. Emmanuel had to sleep in the reclining chair next to my hospital bed for the night. We watched Love Island and fell asleep early.

The next day I was woken up by the nurses at 7 a.m. and was given medication to prevent acid reflux during the cesarean. My blood pressure and oxygen saturation levels were taken and we were again left alone to wait. At 8 a.m. the nurses changed shifts and we were visited once more. This time we were told we would be going to theater today at some point. Today would be my baby's birthday. I liked the date it had fallen on, which was a weird thing to focus on. Somehow February 19th would not have suited Zach and likewise the 17th. The 18th was a good day for him to be born. Then we waited and waited again. We messaged family and friends to let them know what was going on but truthfully, we were floating around with no idea.

At lunchtime, I was given some compression socks to put on and antibacterial wipes to wash with, along with a gown. I got washed up, dressed and sat on the bed so that Emmanuel could help with my compression socks. Trust me when I say there is no easy way to put on a pair of compression socks. It took about half an hour to get on just one sock. My feet were so swollen and the socks, of course, were so tight that the task became a hilarious event of pushing and pulling. It did not help matters that I had not shaved my legs for months—added friction.

Finally, with the socks on, we were called to theater. It was literally a knock on the door and let's go. First, we were taken to another room in another ward. This would be the room that I would come to afterwards for recovery. We lugged all of our bags and bits and pieces across. I set up my bottle of water and tablet ready on the table for afterwards. Then we sat taking in the view overlooking the London Eye. We took some last photos of the two of us dressed in my gown and Emmanuel in his hospital scrubs. The knock on the door came again and off we went. We walked down the corridor to the operating theater.

The theater was not what I expected. We walked in through two sets of doors to a green-colored room and that was it. It was right off the main corridor, almost as if you could stumble into it. I sat on the bed and was given a chair to rest my feet on. My blood pressure and vitals were all checked before we started, and then the procedure was explained to me. I had a cannula inserted into my hand for drugs to be administered then a fluid drip was set up. I was given a pillow to lean over and hug onto. The anesthesiologist then cleaned and numbed the skin on my back. She pushed between two of my vertebrae with her fingers for a while before finding the correct spot. She then inserted the needle and administered the spinal block. I could feel it, but I felt more pressure than pain. Almost straight away my legs went tingly and I felt sick. I was helped to lie down before I lost any more feeling.

Emmanuel was given a chair so that he could sit by my head the whole time. The anesthesiologist stood on the other side of me. From start to finish I could not have asked for anybody more kind or professional to take care of me. My gown was lifted to be used as a screen and a blanket was placed over my lower half. Then came the part I had been truly dreading and I mean that—the catheter. My legs were moved by the nurses and the catheter was inserted. I had no idea about any of it of course but I knew what they were doing as they were talking and telling me as they went. I found this to be the worst part. It still makes my tummy feel funny just thinking about it.

The anesthesiologist used a cold spray to check I was numb all over before anything began. Once she was happy that I could not feel anything anywhere, we were ready. I was giving her detailed feedback, "Well I know you are there, but it doesn't feel cold."

I'm sure she was used to this. I was concentrating so hard in case I could feel anything, but I couldn't at all. They do explain to you that they take away the pain but not the sensations so you will feel movement. They said it would be like rummaging in a handbag—nice analogy!

There I was, Emmanuel holding my hand, everything numb and ready to go, but the surgeon was nowhere to be found. The anesthesiologist stepped up and called someone to sort it out. She was efficient and assertive. It was just what was needed at the time. Once the surgeon entered, he took a moment to introduce himself before a proper screen was put up. I could no longer see anything except the blue fabric, Emmanuel and the anesthesiologist.

Before the surgery started, my blood pressure dropped and I began feeling sick. The anesthesiologist gave me drugs to counteract this and I felt better almost right away. I was a bit shaky but this was just the adrenaline in my body. Then the procedure started. Within minutes we heard them saying, "We can see the baby's feet and bum." They all laughed as he pooed on his way out.

Then we heard the most beautiful sound I have ever heard in my life— my baby boy crying as he was lifted out of me. The anesthesiologist took my phone and snapped loads of pictures for us. Thanks to her, I have a picture sequence of the most amazing moments—Zach's bum being lifted out, his face appearing, his cord being cut, his screaming face and long body stretched out as they lay him across my legs. Zach was taken aside for a few moments to be checked and wrapped in a blanket before being brought over to me. Because of the poo, he had to go straight to the NICU (Neonatal Intensive Care Unit) but I had a few brief moments with him placed next to my face. He reached out and grabbed at my face, as if he knew who I was and was asking to stay with me—but soon, too soon— he was gone.

Emmanuel kissed and hugged me and told me well done before he left with our baby. I was so adamant that he stayed with our son that I'm sure I was practically shouting it. I was alone in a room full of strangers, but the most wonderful strangers. The nurses chatted to me and kept me calm as they started to stitch me back up. I thought I would feel sad because my baby and my partner had both just left, but I felt pretty good.

As they stitched me back up, the student nurse and the anesthesiologist kept up the conversation. "Is this your first baby? Did you know you were having a boy?"—questions that I would soon get very used to hearing and answering. I asked how the stitching was going and was told they were nearly done. I asked again, "No, I mean what layer are they on?" The anesthesiologist paused before answering and telling me there were three to go—fat and two skin. I told her I had watched a video online about how the surgery was done. She laughed and nodded.

The surgeon leaned over the screen and informed me that he had knotted the stitches on the outside and they would likely need cutting off later. The midwives would do this. He said good bye and disappeared off. The nurses cleaned me and gave me a painkiller in the form of a suppository. I had no idea and wished they hadn't told me. I was leaned onto my side so they could clean the blood off me fully and then move me onto a traveling bed.

That was it. I thanked everybody as I was wheeled out of theater and down the corridor into my room. It was over. I had given birth to our son and he was beautiful. The feeling is something I cannot explain—hearing him cry and seeing his face for the first time. Something inside my heart moved for him. We stayed with Zach in hospital for a further six weeks whilst he had two heart surgeries.

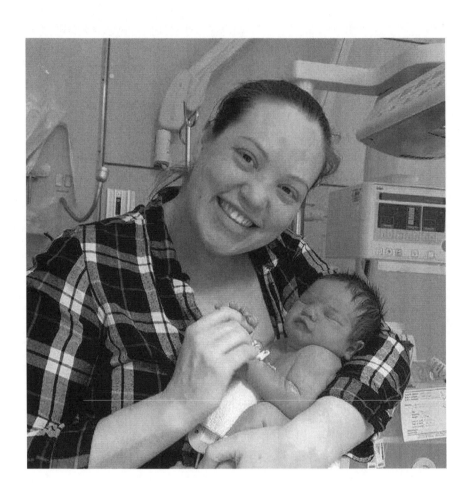

Charlotte, United Kingdom:

** Content warning for weight loss and disordered eating.

My birth story is a positive one against the odds. I am small-fat, have PCOS and only ovulate once in a blue moon when the planets are correctly aligned or something equally rare. To access the fertility treatment we needed to conceive, I had shrunk and punished my body and brain until I was a shell of a person sitting in an eating disorder clinic... but BMI access to healthcare is another story. It is safe to say I was at a pretty low ebb when we discovered I had fallen pregnant between fertility protocols.

Since I fell pregnant between fertility treatment cycles, it was deemed a "natural" pregnancy—despite the fact that my hormones were only kicking in because I had injected so many other people's hormones into me. We went from almost daily intrusive monitoring to being on our own until the twelve-week scan. Panic definitely set in a little.

Knowing that my brain was not in a great place, I had to do something to maintain my recovery and not go into a blind panic over labor and birth. I had discovered a love of complementary therapies and meditative practice during our fertility treatment, so when I learned about the idea of hypnobirthing, I was sold. I started listening to daily hypnotherapy sessions at bedtime. It was relaxing and helped build a positive attitude towards my forthcoming birth. My weight had recovered to almost its set point and with my PCOS diagnosis came blood glucose testing and various eyeroll comments from doctors and midwives. Unfortunately, there is a weight bias in maternity care but my eating disorder treatment and progressively more angry feminist stand to "smash the diet industry" kept me strong.

I was six days over my due date when contractions started over Easter weekend. The ideas I'd learned through hypnobirthing were to prepare for the unexpected and to believe in my own innate inner strength and ability to birth—whatever birth looked like. I had seen some fantastic positive cesarean birth stories, home births, drug-free, drugged up...all kinds shown in a positive light and thank goodness I had!

My total labor was over sixty hours with active labor of around three hours. I started with contractions six minutes apart and the damn things did not get closer together. But here's the thing—it was manageable all the way through. After twenty-four hours, I started to get a bit anxious that things were not moving along, popped into the hospital to get checked out and was sent home again to calm the hell down. I went into the "zoooone": TENS* machine on, clary sage on a hanky, zen up to the eyeballs.

Time no longer had meaning so you will have to excuse sketchy time frames for the next part. The midwives took me and popped me into a room on the maternity suite where they clocked straight away that I was hypnobirthing. They were excited because they all loved hypnobirths apparently. I honestly believe if it was not for them advocating for me and my zen-ness that my birth story would be very different.

Baby was monitored every half hour, which I found reassuring, and I had a few checks. Having had the world and her mother looking up my hoo-ha during fertility treatment, I had a rather blasé attitude towards people taking a look up there. The words "The more the merrier," may have been uttered at some point. I chilled in the birthing pool for about thirty seconds and then realized I was too short to sit comfortably and keep my arm out of the water. I had a cannula for fluids because I kept puking and antibiotics because I was group B strep positive. Once I got out of the pool, a consultant started snooping.

Things were not moving fast enough for his liking and they started bombarding us with options. This is the point where I thank the midwives, my husband and the fact the hypnobirthing had kept me calm enough to advocate for myself. I was not about to do anything suggested without understanding my options.

At that point the midwife decided we were going to work together to get baby out before the consultant did his next rounds. They broke my waters with an amnihook and honestly, by this point, I was well up for it! Shortly after, the involuntary pushing started—it was finally active labor. The pushing and birth part felt like it took about twenty minutes, but apparently it was a couple of hours. Damn it was satisfying to be finally getting my kiddo out!

At this point dignity as I knew it flew out the window. I mean literally; I was boiling hot and demanded a window be opened—only the window faced another window, which appeared to be the nurse's break room. So I was grunting and mooing and omming (which I learned in pregnancy yoga) and the midwife had a flimsy white sheet over my legs to cover me. I remember saying, "You're looking right up my fanny. Why do I need a sheet to cover the front part?"—so that got ditched. I am pretty sure there was a male nurse who did not enjoy his cuppa during his break.

A big push and the head came out—ooh that burned! Another push and plop, he was out. My 9 lb little munchkin all covered in his own poop and goop. I was elated, I had actually done it. After years of hearing the horror story that was my mum giving birth to me, I had broken that trauma with an unconventional but positive and empowered experience. Oxytocin high!

I took the injection to get the placenta out quicker. I had planned to do it the natural way but I'd had quite enough of laboring at that point. I got a few stitches while they checked over the little chap, who had been swimming around in meconium, so he needed a bit of monitoring. He was so red, scrunched up and cute. The midwives at the hospital were all trained aromatherapists so one mixed up a concoction of lavender oil and water for me to use as a sitz bath, which was heaven.

My birth wasn't easy and it wasn't what I thought it would be, but it was quite an experience. I was privileged that in being a small-fat, I was just under the radar for being consultant-led. Had that been the case I think I would have hugely benefited from a doula being present to help advocate for me.

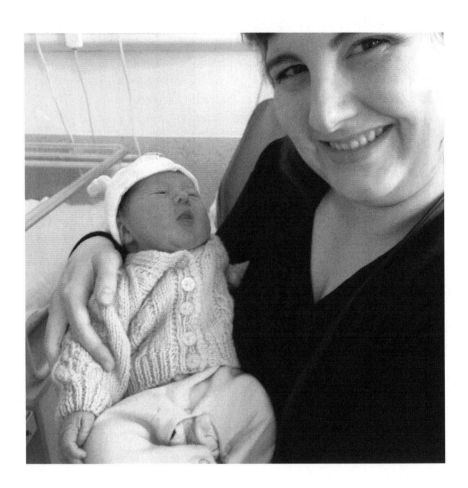

Chelsy Meyer, United States:

I had never heard of moon water before. My friends are a mystic bunch who love crystals and living their life by the moon phases. While I am not as connected to this as they are, I consider myself to be a spiritual-enough person.

On the night that I learned about moon water, I was five months pregnant with my son. He is my miracle, conceived with the help of science after my husband and I dealt with fertility issues. It was a full moon in summer and my friends explained that moon water could be created by leaving a cup of water out overnight to be charged by the full moon. Afterwards, you can use the water to drink, bathe, paint with and more.

It is true that the moon can manipulate water—that is how we have ocean tides—so I thought the magic of it all was interesting. I filled a tiny mason jar and took it home to soak in the moon's power overnight. I took it with me into the bathroom and poured the freezing contents over my swollen belly during my morning shower.

Four months later, on the night of the winter solstice, my moon baby was born. I love this celestial coincidence. Whether I believe it is truly connected or not, I love the beautiful themes surrounding the sun and moon, and how they translate to rebirth and light.

On the morning of the solstice, I walked into the hospital for my planned induction. The plan was to start the induction, get the epidural and hopefully have my baby vaginally. I really wanted to be flexible while focusing on the end goal—for us both to be healthy at the end of it all, no matter how that had to happen.

The first few hours of labor were largely uneventful. I was given Pitocin and I walked around when I began to feel uncomfortable. I dilated to 5 cm pretty easily but then hit a plateau. We decided to release my waters to get things moving—and boy did it! The amount of fluid that came out was absurd and I was given a lawn-chair-sized pad to use. While the first few hours were largely pain-free, this was when my luck ran out.

The pain that came on was immense and arrived like a tsunami over my body. Walking did not help. Sitting did not help. Cursing did not help. Crying did not help. Nothing helped. I used every ounce of strength I had to get through each contraction, only to be hit with another wave a few minutes later. I cried into my husband's shirt and tried to fight off the feeling of weakness as the pain rocked through my body. I decided it was time to get the epidural.

In hindsight, I got it too early. I don't remember pain when getting the epidural—I only remember the strength it took to sit still through each contraction as they put the needle into my spine. I held onto my husband and silently cried, digging down as deep as I could for the willpower to sit still. Thankfully, the pain subsided. Soon I could not move my stomach muscles enough to cough. No amount of concentration could even move a toe. I was so excited that I wouldn't be able to feel my baby come out at all.

I tried to sleep, but mostly just had liquids and watched movies. While I didn't want anyone there for labor except my husband, my dad came to see me before things really started happening. Seeing him felt comforting, like I was doing something exciting and not scary. Although I didn't feel cold, I started shivering pretty violently while he was visiting. The nurse told us the shivering was a sign of transition so I texted my doula.

The power a doula has is amazing. I felt comfortable enough with her beforehand, as we had met a few times during my pregnancy. We had gone over my birth plan, and I'd had the opportunity to ask questions. In my hospital room my doula brought with her so much strength and calm. She lit some candles and played low music. She did not overwhelm me, but stayed close by. I felt so much better once she arrived, but I soon began to feel pain again.

They gave me a peanut ball and told me to try to get some sleep, but my anxiety, the pain and having to be shifted every fifteen minutes meant that didn't happen. I felt pain, looked at the monitors and saw that my pain was coinciding with contractions. I kept hitting the button to release more pain medication within the epidural, but it didn't seem to be working. I could only hit the button every fifteen minutes, but I was hitting it like you hit a crosswalk button—you know hitting the button repeatedly won't make the light change any quicker, but you do it anyway just to feel like you are doing something. I was soon moving my legs around the peanut ball on my own.

At 8 p.m., twelve hours after being induced, they checked my cervix again and realized I was at 10 cm. It was time to start pushing! My epidural was wearing off and the pain was there no matter how much I hit the button, but it was time. I knew I had to do this without adequate pain relief.

I lay on my back, held my thighs and my doula counted to eight while I tried to feel how to push. That poor woman must have counted to eight a billion times! At first I didn't know what I was doing. I was trying to feel how to push but thought I wasn't doing it correctly. I felt insecure as everyone watched my body pushing and congratulated me for pushing hard. I held my thighs and tried to coordinate breathing and pushing when they told me to. Sometimes I did it wrong, and other times I questioned whether I was pushing at the right point of a contraction. Eventually they brought me a birthing bar to hold onto for leverage instead of my thighs.

It hurt—a lot. I could feel pressure; I could feel pain. I was pushing but I did not feel like anything was happening. I just knew I wasn't doing it right. Finally, I asked if I could get on my knees.

The fact that I got onto my knees on my own, despite having an epidural, tells you all you need to know about how well the medicine was working. I could feel my legs just fine. I draped my body over the back of the bed, grabbed the bar that was back there and pushed as hard as I could. Now I could feel progress. I don't remember exactly how the pain felt, but I do remember that there was a lot of it. I thought *I won't be able to do this!* It was funny that only a few hours before I'd been excited about the prospect of having a baby without pain.

I remember discussing pain during my childbirth class with a midwife and consultations with my doula. We discussed the difference between suffering and the pain that leads to progress in labor. It was hard to remember the difference when I was pushing and actually feeling the pain. It was easy to get lost in how much it hurt—but remembering that this was pain with a purpose was paramount for my mental stamina.

As my baby got closer and closer, the insecurity over people seeing my body push and feeling embarrassed was gone. My head poured sweat into my hair. I screamed and cried as I pushed with the contractions. I tried to visualize waves washing in and out. My husband brought me water to drink and a cold washcloth for my head. My eyes stayed closed, but I was so happy to have him there at the head of my bed and not the foot so I did not feel alone.

My doula kept counting and counting. She asked me what I was thinking, and I told her, "Everything worth having is hard." She was proud of me for keeping my mindset in a positive place. I felt like I'd been pushing for so long, but my doctor wasn't there yet. I thought that must mean I wasn't close to giving birth. *Why isn't my baby coming?* As I laid draped over the bed, I tried to focus so I did not break down. I tried to remember how small this window of time would be in the large expanse of my baby's life—how in a few hours it would all be over. I started to feel desperate. I had been pushing for over two hours. I eventually started crying and saying, "I can't do this!"

Then a blip of memory popped into my head. In my consultations with my doula she had said, "When women start to say 'I can't do this,' I know the baby is about to come."

My doctor still hadn't arrived. I was too afraid to ask them if I was making progress because I was in so much pain. If they had told me that my baby was not coming despite all the agony and pushing, I would have given up. It would have broken me. I still felt that if my obstetrician was not there, my baby was not near. Little did I know that they had contacted her about my son's heart rate, which was a little high. She was on her way.

I kept pushing with all of my might while on my knees, but it was hard for my nurses to see what was going on. Finally, I heard my doula say, "Oh my God, that's his head!" They had no idea the baby was so close because of my position. They ran to get the on-call delivery doctor and said, "Chelsy, the baby is coming—the on-call delivery doctor is going to have to deliver your baby." I did not care who was going to deliver the baby at this point. I was desperate to GET HIM OUT!

Just then, my obstetrician ran in the door. She scrambled to get her gloves, boots and gown on. I was facing the other way, but I heard the commotion. They tried to get me to breathe with tiny, fast breaths as I finished pushing to avoid tearing, but I did not listen. I gave it all I had and pushed as hard as I could. I felt my baby leave my body and I heard him cry as the room exploded with excitement. Once his head was out, his shoulders were not a problem and he arrived at 10:38 p.m.

I wish I could explain the relief. All the pain, all the screaming, all the fear and all the doubt washed away in a wave of solace. My body sank like a deflated balloon. My eyes stayed closed and my head dropped while my hands and arms released tension. My hair both hung in my face and stuck to my forehead. My baby was here. I could hear him crying. It was over. I had done it.

I whispered, "I'll be there in a second, baby—I just need a minute," but I'm sure no one heard me.

My husband cried into my hair, "Our baby is here!"

I gathered my strength and flipped myself over but there were so many wires. I felt a new one hindering me and realized it was the umbilical cord. I will never forget the feel of it against my legs. I opened my birthing gown and my warm, creamy, pink baby was placed on my chest. I looked at him and said, "We did it, baby! Happy birthday."

I looked at him without surprise, like I always knew this was what he would look like. He was here—my moon baby. It was the single most spectacular thing I had ever done. I was overwhelmed with appreciation for my body, my doctor, my nurses, my doula and my husband. I wanted to hug everyone. My husband held onto me while I held the baby, and I got to see him become a dad. His eyes were glossy as he gazed at our baby, and I loved him even more than I thought I could.

The next few hours were a blur. My husband cut the umbilical cord and I was stitched. I got the baby to latch and he nursed for an hour. He was measured, weighed and wrapped up. As we nestled into our room, I stared out into the dark winter morning through the window. The world was so still, and my baby slept while holding onto me. I never felt so important, so protective, so full of purpose. I was his home—his safe place. Despite the exhaustion and the pain, I looked back on what I had just done and felt so much strength in motherhood.

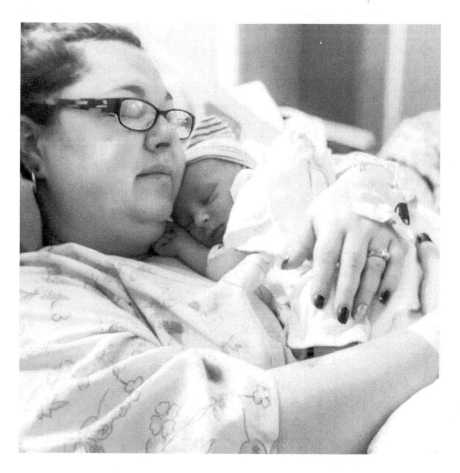

Sophie, Scotland:

*** Content warning for weight stigma in a medical
setting and pregnancy loss.*

Ever since I can remember, I always wanted to have kids. I was obsessed with looking after the younger kids at my childminder's house when I was five, and becoming an aunt at eleven was a dream come true. As I went through my teenage years, the want and need to become a mother just became stronger. I wanted to channel these feelings into something I could turn into a job. I was accepted onto a midwifery course; it was the perfect career.

I packed up my life in the Scottish Borders when I was eighteen and set off an hour north to live in Edinburgh. I stayed in the university halls and had the time of my life studying for my dream career, meeting new friends, drinking and partying.

A year and a half into my midwifery course, I began to wake up severely aching all over. It took me ten minutes to stand and I felt unbelievably fatigued. I thought at first it was the thirteen-hour student placement shifts taking their toll, but I knew deep down it was much more than that. When I was unable to bend down to the birth pool to support women through their labors, I said enough was enough. I took myself along to the other side of the hospital and went to the Emergency Department—I could barely walk and my hips and knees kept giving way.

They did an x-ray and said there was nothing wrong. They advised me to go to my general practitioner, as it could be some form of arthritis. I went to my doctor, where she looked me up and down and started asking me about my lifestyle. She refused to give me stronger painkillers and advised I probably just needed *to exercise more*. I was absolutely crippled and I honestly could not believe this was said to me. I went home and completely broke down.

A week later my left calf felt extremely heavy and looked very swollen. One of my flatmates was a student nurse and he started reeling off the symptoms of a blood clot. I went to the hospital where an ultrasound confirmed I did in fact have one. I explained all my other pains to the doctor and he was very concerned I had an infection. Little did I know that this conversation would result in a two-week hospital stay to find out what was wrong with me. I was so relieved because I was finally being taken seriously. I might have been young and I might have been fat, but I deserved access to adequate healthcare and answers just as much as the next person.

Very long story short, I was diagnosed with adult-onset Still's disease. This is a very rare condition that is a similar disease to rheumatoid arthritis or lupus. Basically, my immune system goes into overdrive for some unknown reason and attacks my joints, muscles and eventually my organs. My kidneys, liver and heart were all showing signs of strain. Blood clots can be related to Still's disease; if I had not had that first blood clot, who knows where I would have ended up when I was finally taken seriously.

The next year involved a lot of steroids, low-dose chemotherapy and other cocktails of drugs and painkillers. There is no cure for Still's disease, only keeping it at bay and controlling it. I found a drug that worked for me which came in the form of a monthly infusion. It had been amazing, however, the steroids did contribute to additional weight gain. My joints suffered a lot of damage and both my hips have been replaced over the years. I had to give up on my career in midwifery and I completed a degree in finance instead.

I met my husband, Mikey, when I was twenty-one years old. A few months after dating, I took a pregnancy test that came back positive. I was on the copper coil as a hormone-free contraceptive measure so it could not have come as a bigger shock. Although stunned, I was also secretly happy that I would be a mother very soon. I remember smiling to myself in the bathroom before I announced it to Mikey even though I was petrified he would leave me. A dozen positive tests later, it began to sink in slowly and we started making plans.

The pregnancy was not meant to be. Bleeding and a scan, which showed an empty uterus, confirmed I was experiencing a loss. I had my coil removed and decided on the implant instead, which would last me three years. I am a firm believer that everything happens for a reason and this baby was not meant for us—we were not ready.

Two and a half years later we were engaged to be married in five months and we felt it was the right time to start trying for children. I could not be more excited to get the implant out—I felt like my life had been leading up to this moment. I bought ovulation sticks and pregnancy tests, completely consuming myself with getting pregnant. Secretly I was very worried that my health issues would prevent pregnancy.

Five months later we were married, but getting my period on our honeymoon in Tenerife was earth-shattering. I was becoming obsessed with getting pregnant and downloaded six different books on how to get pregnant whilst on our honeymoon. I had already had two to three extremely faint lines on pregnancy tests that disappeared a day or two later, more than likely chemical pregnancies. It was a complete rollercoaster of emotions. I got easily sucked into the copious amount of online resources which basically said that fat people do not get pregnant—especially if they were my size. My husband and I wanted a baby so badly, and I saw how he was just as hurt as me with every negative test.

We arrived back from our honeymoon with only one month until Christmas. I put the ovulation sticks, the ovulation apps and fertility lube to one side and concentrated on a strategy from one of the books—we did the deed every second day with no other help.

I had a small amount of bleeding on January 1st—a sure sign that my period was imminent. A small part of me started to hope that maybe, just maybe, this could be the long-awaited implantation bleeding I had learned about. I took a pregnancy test at home the following day and an extremely faint line was there. I did not get excited, in fact, I did the opposite. I thought this too would end with another chemical pregnancy. I told my husband not to get excited as it would probably end in disappointment.

The test line got darker and darker over the next two days whenever I tested. We finally let go and started to get excited that maybe I really was pregnant. This feeling was sadly overshadowed by the fear that people in bigger bodies are more likely to miscarry. I kept reminding my husband that it was still early days. The fatphobia I had seen online was giving me some seriously bad anxiety.

By eight weeks pregnant, I had already seen a rheumatologist who specialized in young women with arthritis and more specifically, those who are pregnant. We weighed the pros and cons of continuing my infusion medication alongside research on how much of the drug actually crossed the placenta. My infusions were spaced apart as much as possible during my pregnancy so it stopped my joints from flaring and minimized exposure to my baby. I was happy with the plan, as were my doctors.

Then it was time for my booking appointment. The midwife and I went through my extensive medical history before the dreaded topic of my weight came up. She wanted to refer me to a specialist metabolic clinic, which I agreed to. She told me my obstetrician would be the one who deals with pregnant people with a higher BMI. I advised her that I would prefer to keep the obstetrician that deals with immune-related conditions instead since I already had some correspondence from her. This was basically denied and she told me she would be referring me to the obstetrician she recommended. I was pissed off that my request had not even been entertained. I had health concerns relating to my Still's disease, not my weight! The obstetrician who knew the most about my pregnancy at that stage would no longer be involved with my care.

Being able to see my baby at the twelve-week scan was amazing. My husband and I were in complete awe of the little person dancing about on the screen in front of us. This happy moment ended when the sonographer advised that she was struggling to get the measurements she needed. She dug harder into my soft belly, signaling the difficulty was due to my size. In the end, she advised that she couldn't do the Down's Syndrome nuchal fold test—where they measure the fluid at the back of baby's neck—which I was fine with.

I had various appointments at the metabolic clinic. My first appointment with the new obstetrician was okay at best and very brief. Being told I would more than likely get gestational diabetes created instant worry. As I was one of the largest expecting mums there, they started to explain how losing weight whilst I was pregnant would be beneficial as well. I ignored that advice, as I did not believe there was a safe or balanced way to approach weight loss during pregnancy.

My twenty-week scan was great; we didn't find out the sex as we wanted a surprise. My glucose tolerance test showed that and behold... I did NOT HAVE GESTATIONAL DIABETES! I did have to stop work at twenty-eight weeks because my knee pain became too intense. This was probably related to pregnancy hormones beginning to relax all my joints and muscles in preparation for labor.

The three growth scans recommended for me always showed baby being on the bigger side—putting major fear into my head again! My last growth scan said the baby was well over 10 lbs and I still had three weeks to go. I began to freak out and started to crave an induction as I became increasingly worried about birthing a massive baby. Looking back now, I am so completely pissed off and genuinely wish I had not had the growth scans. The suspected "big baby" was no grounds for induction. However, the reduced movements I was experiencing were. I was checked often and even though baby was moving away on the monitor, I just could not feel it anymore. The decision was made to begin labor induction at thirty-nine weeks.

I met an anesthetic consultant at one of my last appointments. My birth plan very much involved trying to go into labor myself (which was obviously not happening now), minimal pain relief and absolutely 100 percent avoid a cesarean unless my baby was in danger. The consultant pretty much shut down every single one of those options. The most soul-crushing thing was being advised I should have an epidural as soon as possible to make *their lives easier*. He explained how it could take longer to get the epidural in because of my weight. I felt completely cornered and agreed to add this to my birth plan once the induction had got to the right stage. At this point, I was so fed up with being fat shamed, I just agreed to anything. I just wanted my baby safe on the other side of my supposedly inferior body.

My induction began at thirty-nine weeks and it was slow, to say the least. My baby was clearly not ready to come out. I had the pessary and two rounds of gel* before they said progress had been minimal and they could not release my waters. I was given the option of a cesarean. I couldn't believe it—*is that it?!* Barely any pain or what felt like effort and already I was being told to throw in the towel. "Not a chance," I replied. "I'm not having a cesarean until absolutely necessary."

Only at this point, when they realized how serious I was, did they explore other options. They said I could have a balloon catheter inserted in my cervix to help it dilate, which did not involve any hormones. *Why wasn't I offered this before the cesarean*? I wondered. Cesarean would certainly have been the easier option for them. They had tried for forty-eight hours already to induce me with next to no success.

I had the balloon catheter inserted and had the absolute time of my life on gas and air. I went back to the ward and boy, did those contractions start! I was screaming and swearing in a four-bed antenatal ward while grabbing the bed rails. I was left with no pain relief for what felt like hours. The consultant finally came back and agreed to remove some of the water in the balloon. This made such a difference and even though I was still uncomfortable, it was much better.

My husband left and the monitor showed some contractions, which I was pleased with. The midwives came in at 5 a.m. and said one of my blood results came back showing my body was starting to struggle a bit. They wanted to take me to the labor ward to break my waters. It was finally happening! I was so excited to get things moving.

---

*   Synthetic prostaglandin gel may be applied during the induction process to help soften and thin the cervix. A pessary looks much like a small tampon and may be used internally to apply prostaglandin gel to the cervix.

My husband arrived back just in time for my waters being released at 3 cm dilated. The oxytocin drip was started and my contractions had begun. I told my husband to get something to eat while my epidural was placed, as I thought it would be quick. It was not, unfortunately, and it took a few tries before it was sited properly. I felt so alone and scared, but I puffed away on the gas and air in an attempt to drown out the commotion behind me.

The next four hours ticked away nicely with the contractions showing on the monitor and my pain pretty much non-existent. They examined me and I was so hopeful I had progressed a good amount. "Two centimeters," the consultant advised.

2cm? How could I be 2 cm when I was 3 cm four hours ago? They explained that when they remove the balloon catheter, the cervix may go slack and close a bit. I was devastated. I just knew at that point I would need a cesarean. My limited knowledge from my midwifery placements years ago was just sitting in the back of my mind. I carried on laboring for another four hours with, as I thought, no change in dilation. The baby was having small decelerations in it's heart rate now so the time had come. The doctor sat on my bed and tried to break the news to me as gently as she could. I burst into tears when I was told I would be having a cesarean. At this stage, I was content with the fact that I had done everything possible with the information I had to try having my baby vaginally. The surgery risks were explained to me, including the heightened risks for someone of my size. I signed the consent forms knowing my three-day induction was soon coming to an end.

My husband joined me in the operating theater donned in his blue scrubs. I was hooked up to machines and drips from every angle before the surgery began. Even though it was classed as an emergency cesarean, it was strangely calm. All of the staff were amazing and in good spirits. After a lot of tugging and pulling the consultant said, "Hello darling!" and just like that, our baby was out screaming the world down! My birth plan stated that Mikey would announce the sex. When the staff asked him to, he was crying so much he couldn't see what it was. One of the doctors whispered "girl" and Mikey said it through his broken voice. We had a beautiful baby girl.

The midwives whisked her off to clean her up and she was absolutely perfect. We named her Amelia Grace and she weighed in at 8 lbs 11 oz. She was born three days before forty weeks and she was a long way from the 10 lbs+ she was predicted to weigh at my antenatal appointment three weeks earlier.

I had a proper opportunity to hold Amelia in recovery and she latched on to breastfeed straight away. I was so happy. I finally had everything I ever wanted.

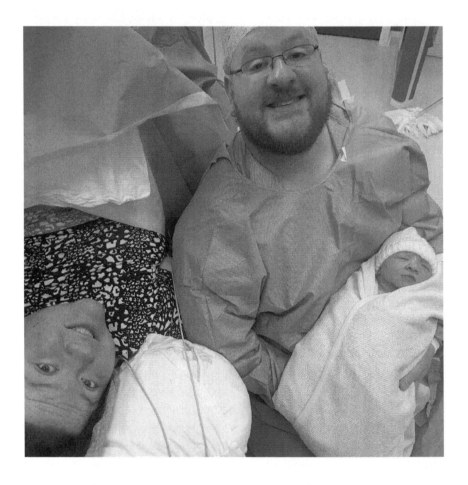

Annika, Ireland:

It was 12:20 a.m. on the night of June 22nd, 2018 when our third baby let us know that she was ready to come into this world. After nearly two weeks of my body preparing itself with practice surges, things were now moving!

After a less-than-ideal birthing experience with our second baby, we knew very early on in the pregnancy that we wanted a home birth this time around. This made it all the more special when surges started, as we did not have to think about preparations for having our two other children taken care of, or when to go into hospital. Although home births are gaining in popularity, we were frequently met with disbelief and outright opposition when we mentioned our plans. As a result, we actively decided to only allow positive thoughts and stories into our space and discarded the rest. We felt informed, relaxed and so excited for the birth.

After going to bed and getting some sleep, the surges increased in intensity in the early morning hours. I got up but was still very comfortable, so I asked my partner to stay in bed. He would need his energy for later in the day! I informed our midwife and a friend who had offered to look after our three-year-old daughter and two-year-old son. I then busied myself around the house for a while. It promised to be a wonderful day—the midwife and my friend arrived, everyone got up, pancakes were made and jokes were told. All the while, monitoring continued in a completely relaxed and non-invasive way. It just seemed like such a normal thing to have a birth. The support of a wonderful midwife and friends made it possible.

A short while later, the surges got stronger and started to take all of my attention. My partner knew exactly what to do and how to support me through touch, affirmations and key words. Things continued to progress very quickly. Our daughter insisted on being present for the birth as she jumped around the bedroom, excitedly waiting for the baby to arrive.

Without so much as a single push and in three final surges, baby Flynne Isabella came into this world at 10:31 a.m., weighing 10 lbs l6 oz. She was calm, relaxed and full of life. To this day she is very much how she was born—a thriving, very relaxed child, who knows her mind.

Mikaylea Glaeser, United States:

Sunday October 25th I woke up with a backache. I was thirty-eight weeks and one day pregnant and twenty years old. I told my husband Ethan, "My back really hurts today," and he asked if I thought it was labor. I said no and did not think much of it as we prepared to go to my mom's house for a family day. I sat on her exercise ball and did a puzzle most of the morning. My back continued to ache—the intensity growing like a wave building up and crashing into rocks. I started to feel some pressure and tightness in the front as well and decided to text the birth phone and give my midwives a heads up. The student midwife texted me back and asked me to check back in with her in an hour.

By the time an hour rolled around, I was very uncomfortable and could not talk through the contractions anymore. I called the student midwife and said labor was picking up and we should probably head to the birth center soon. The next few contractions got very intense, and I squatted in my mom's living room moaning, trying to relieve the pain in my back. Ethan put our things in the car, and we left our fifteen-month-old at my mom's for the time being. We stopped by our house to grab the new baby's car seat and my birth bags. I could not sit in the car; it was so painful. I was on my hands and knees, moaning and yelling through the contractions.

We arrived at the birth center and I labored for quite a while with the TENS unit on my back. I started feeling super shaky and nauseous, like I could be in transition. I asked to get in the tub and the midwives started filling it right away. I got in and then my midwife asked if she could check me—she felt like something was off. I said yes. She checked me and I was only 3 cm dilated. They wanted me out of the tub, which I reluctantly did. The student midwife helped me do lots of positional work to bring baby down and help my cervix dilate more.

I labored for twelve hours and asked to have a chiropractor come adjust me—the pain in my back had become unbearable and I hoped it would help me progress. My back felt better immediately following the adjustment, but my labor slowed. Within four hours, my contractions had completely stopped and all the pressure in my pelvis was gone. Everything stopped and even my brain felt different. I asked for another internal exam to check dilation and if I could go home. I was at 4 cm so the midwives said it was fine to return home.

I thought showering and sleeping in my own bed might help spur things along but nothing happened. I hardly had a single contraction for days. On October 28th, I had five to eight contractions the entire day but nothing notable, strong or consistent. I went to bed with no expectations of having a baby anytime soon. I had already thought he would wait to be born until at least the 30th because my mom was seeing an oncologist on the 29th. I woke up at 11:30 p.m. on the 28th, feeling weird. My pad was wet and mucusy, and I felt decent contractions. I went to the bathroom and decided to take a shower. The contractions were now strong, intense and very close together. Within minutes they were so strong that I was getting loud and decided to wake Ethan. It felt like I had been in the shower for an hour at least, however I discovered later it was only fifteen minutes. I could barely get the ten feet from the shower to the bed to wake Ethan—that was how intense everything felt. I squatted with a contraction and tried to grab his foot to wake him. He did not wake easily and all I could get out was, "We've got to go, we've got to go!"

Finally, he woke up and figured out what was happening. I called the photographer, my mom and then the birth center phone. All I could get out is, "This is it! It really, really hurts!" One of the students answered and told me to head to the birth center right away.

We got to the birth center just after midnight. I could barely talk or walk—the intensity was so high. I asked if they could check me and I was almost 6 cm dilated. I labored on the ball and my hands and knees for a while, but I could not focus through the intensity. I begged to get in the water. The midwives started filling the tub, but I knew it would take between twenty and thirty minutes for it to be full enough for me to get in. I got into my own head a bit and started crying, "I can't do this! It hurts!" I cried over and over.

Ethan rubbed my back and arms and told me he knew I could do it. My midwife came over and stopped me—"Get out of your head. Put your doula hat on. Coach yourself like you would a client. You can do this. You were made for this."

It was exactly what I needed to hear. I paced around the room, quickly trying to escape the pain. I cried for my mom and asked them to tell her to come in. I got in the tub, and it made everything so much more manageable.

Labor was still intense but I was much more able to focus. I instinctively scooped water on top of my belly during contractions and the students started taking turns using a pitcher to pour water on me instead. It helped the pain even more at that point. My mom came and I was able to get into a good mindset as soon as I saw her. I kept asking if it was real, if I was really going to have a baby this time. Everyone kept assuring me that this was real and I was going to meet my baby soon. The intensity made it feel like hours had passed. I was starting to feel so much pressure and asked to be checked again. "Am I almost done? Please tell me I'm almost done," I said.

My midwife told me, "You're almost done—you're so close. You're over 8 cm!"

At that point, I knew I could do it. *I can do this. I'm almost done. I can do this.* I felt determination enter me instead of the defeat and discouragement I had been feeling. Within two contractions, my body started pushing. The pressure was so intense, but I focused hard and tried to surrender to the feeling and just relax everything. I reached down and I said, "I can feel him, his head is right there. He's almost here!"

I was so relieved. My midwife asked if I wanted her to support my perineum, and if she could check for a nuchal cord when his head came. I agreed to both. I could feel his head crowning and I yelled trying to relax and let my body slowly stretch through the burning.

"Oh my gosh! I think you're going to have an en caul baby!" the midwives said. I could not believe it! I was so excited. Another contraction happened and the midwife said, "Now is the time if you want to catch your baby!" I reached down to feel his head and moments later his shoulders and body were born. I brought him up to my chest—he was here.

My baby boy was born in water, still in the caul and caught by my own hands. I was shocked when they announced it was 2:26 a.m. I thought for sure it was seven or eight in the morning. My son was so alert and aware immediately, looking right into my eyes. It was the most beautiful experience and so much more peaceful than my first birth. He weighed 7 lbs 3 oz of absolute perfection. All I could do was cry with happiness and say over and over that I loved him.

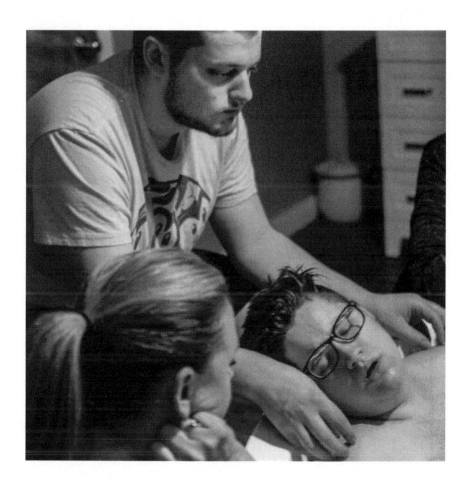

Sam, UK:

My birth experience began with a membrane sweep on a Wednesday afternoon. My contractions started the following morning at 5 a.m., carried on until 2 p.m. and then stopped. The next day some of my mucus plug released and the contractions started again at about 2 p.m., They were more regular this time and getting stronger. My cousin lent me her TENS machine, which I found so helpful. It didn't stop the pain but it certainly took the edge off.

I called the labor ward at 8 p.m. and they confirmed I would need to wait a bit longer until contractions were coming every two to three minutes before I would be admitted. I could not take the intensity of my contractions anymore at 3 a.m., so I called them again. I was admitted at 5 a.m. and was told I was 5 cm dilated following an internal examination. My waters had partly released so they broke them the rest of the way and put an internal fetal monitor onto my baby's head. The wireless monitor they usually used was not working very well. They offered me gas and air, which was amazing, and I carried on with that.

At 9:30 a.m., I felt the need to start pushing, however, they realized my son was in a slightly turned position when they checked me. His heart rate was also dropping during my contractions, which led to loads of people suddenly entering the room. I was told my baby needed to come out now and the staff were going to help with use of a ventouse.

They managed to get him most of the way with the vacuum, but they ultimately had to use forceps for the last couple of contractions. I cannot tell you the pressure I felt with those forceps in. It certainly was the worst part of my labor. My beautiful baby boy arrived at 10:50 a.m. and was brought to the NICU for further monitoring.

I had the injection to deliver my placenta afterward, which was out in a few minutes, and went on to have a lovely cuppa and toast that the midwives brought me. Although the end of my birth was more challenging than I imagined, I still look at it as a positive.

Caitlyn PW Jones, United States:

Ayla was born March 28th, 2020 at thirty-seven weeks. There was a lot of uncertainty surrounding her birth but ultimately, I had a positive birth experience.

After being on modified bed rest for six months, I was sent to the hospital from my thirty-seven-week doctor's appointment. I was to be induced immediately due to signs of intrauterine growth restriction (IUGR). By 4:30 p.m. that day, I was checked in at the hospital and Cervidil was placed internally in order to begin softening my cervix. I was prepared for it to be a journey. My husband, Eric, and I had packed our hospital bags a few weeks earlier. I packed my headphones and had my birth affirmations ready on my phone. I had my K-pop playlist cued up for extra motivation when needed. I was told to rest as much as possible but the stronger contractions and nervous energy made it near impossible to sleep that night.

The nurse took out the Cervidil and I was started on an IV of Pitocin to kickstart my labor Friday morning. That afternoon, the doctor on call checked me and I was 1 cm dilated, 50 percent effaced and baby's head was down low. I knew I had to be patient but after being told my baby was not growing fast enough and that my placenta was slowly failing at its job—I just wanted her to be safely in my arms. Around 4 p.m., the doctor checked me again and I was 3 cm dilated. With permission, the doctor released my waters. I had been experiencing prodromal labor for weeks, but after my waters were broken my contractions intensified. As they wracked my body with a promise of never letting go, I knew I had to breathe and shift my focal point.

During each contraction I recited my three birth affirmations:

> I can do anything for sixty seconds
> This surge is not stronger than me because it is a part of me
> Each wave brings me closer to meeting my daughter

I was able to deliver vaginally as planned but ended up getting an epidural because of complications. Ayla's heart rate kept dropping during labor and I needed to stay completely still to monitor her. Since I have some health issues, mainly fibromyalgia, moving and changing labor positions often was an intricate part of my natural pain management plan. After much deliberation, I decided to get the epidural for the safety of my baby. The anesthesiologist was so sweet. He said I was very calm while he administered the epidural and he knew I would make a good mother.

Around 9:30 p.m. that night, when I was almost 5 cm, I threw up. It was not much because I was only allowed ice chips and two red ice pops when my blood sugar was low. Having gestational diabetes, I received regular finger sticks during and after labor. My nurse that night was amazing. She stayed by my side monitoring Ayla's heartbeat and kept my peanut ball between my numb legs. I finally told her I felt pressure and she was a little skeptical, but she went to look. She then looked up and asked, "Where did your husband go? It's time to have this baby!"

My husband had stepped out to update his family and I had to call him to hurry back. I went from 4 to 10 cm dilated in an hour and a half and started pushing at 10:45 p.m. After the first few pushes, my nurse and Eric said they could already see her head! My contractions were still pretty far apart, at every eight minutes, so I would snooze between pushing. My nurse instructed me on several pushing techniques until I found one that was comfortable. The doctor came in after a while and Ayla begrudgingly came out soon after. She was 5 lbs 8 oz.

Three hours later, Ayla had breastfed twice, and our little family was all settled in the postpartum wing upstairs. Eric and Ayla fell asleep as soon as the nurse turned the lights out. I stayed up thanking Jehovah God for such a healthy and beautiful baby girl. All my struggles were well worth this gift lying beside me and I would, without hesitation, do it all again.

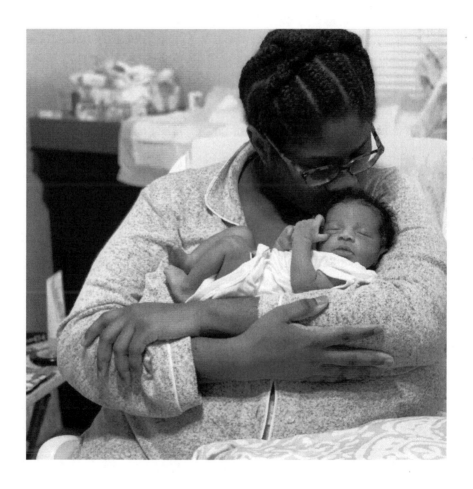

Erika, Canada:

My pregnancy journey felt like a rollercoaster of emotions. It looked nothing like I had originally envisioned and looking back, I would 100 percent do it again!

My anxiety kicked in before even getting pregnant, as I had read multiple articles suggesting that people with a high BMI have a harder time getting pregnant. A doctor informed me of the same. I was hoping I would get pregnant without any real hassle, yet the doctor's voice played on repeat like a bad song in my head. The joke was on him though because following my IUD removal a month later, I got pregnant within weeks!

Once pregnant, I knew I wanted a size-friendly healthcare provider. I decided to pursue midwifery care after hearing many positive experiences from friends. I ended up connecting with a lovely midwife who allowed me to feel safe, ask questions and reminded me that my body was capable.

Halfway through my pregnancy, my midwife told me she would be sending me for some bloodwork. This led to my diagnosis of gestational diabetes, and I was heartbroken. I felt as if I were feeding into the "fat lady pregnancy stats" and my pregnancy would probably go exactly as the non-supportive doctor had dictated. Once the shock of my diagnosis kicked in and tears were shed, I bought a few cook books, joined some online groups and realized that people of all sizes can have gestational diabetes. Until this diagnosis, I'd had no health challenges in my life and I was going to do whatever I needed to keep my baby safe and healthy.

For me, the one big challenge with this diagnosis was that if I had to start insulin, I would need to transfer care from my midwife to an obstetrician. This was something I definitely wanted to avoid. With lots of discipline and a change in diet (basically being more mindful of the foods I was eating), I was able to keep my blood sugar levels where they needed to be and did not need any insulin during my entire pregnancy.

As I got closer to my due date, my midwife informed me that my baby was "measuring big." She told me that I would need to meet with an obstetrician for a consultation and go for bi-weekly ultrasounds. My baby was measuring in the ninety-eighth percentile from week thirty-two onward. The obstetrician strongly urged me to consider a cesarean because of baby's predicted weight, and, of course, my BMI. Hearing this news enraged me.

I asked some questions which were answered with statements like, "Based on the research, bigger women…"

Although I felt discouraged and uncertain of what to do, I went back to my midwife and asked what she thought, as this was not what I had planned for my birth. After a few more weeks with many tears, contemplation, advice and prayer, I decided if it was going to be safer for my baby, I would do it.

I had the option of trying vaginal birth first but was informed that due to baby's predicted size, there was a high chance it would end in a cesarean due to complications. I was also given the pros and cons for attempting a vaginal birth followed by emergency cesarean—versus going straight for the scheduled cesarean. In the end, I agreed to the planned cesarean.

Now, I know that my story does not seem to be ideal and in all honesty— it was not. I lay down in that operating room, staring at the bright lights above me, spread-eagled on the table with a curtain in front of me, my husband by my side and the room filled with an amazing female medical team. At that moment, the only thing that mattered was my baby. After about twenty minutes of surgery, my beautiful, healthy baby girl was born. They allowed my husband to stand up to see her first and then allowed me to see her before she was quickly weighed and returned to me. She nursed right away and her blood sugar levels were perfect. My little baby girl was healthy, weighing 9 lbs 2 oz. When holding my baby in my arms, nothing else mattered. The gestational diabetes diagnosis, the weekly ultrasounds, the cesarean—it was all worth it.

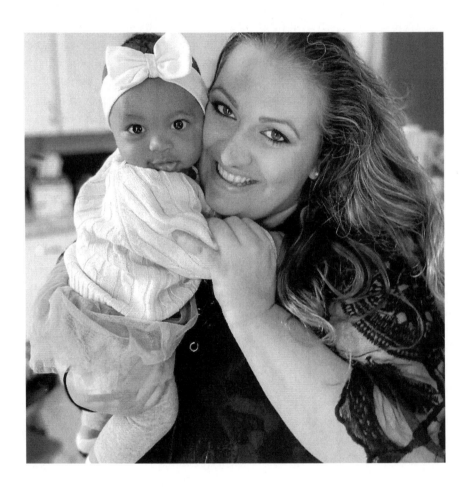

Michelle, United States:

*** *Content warning for obstetric violence.*

I was in a completely different place both physically and emotionally during my second pregnancy. My first child was born just before I turned seventeen and given the eight-year age gap, I had grown up a lot myself. I knew there were many things my husband and I could do to help facilitate a more positive birth experience. We spent months learning about our options for labor and we started to feel more confident and prepared.

Ultimately, what I truly desired was a home birth with few to no interventions, however, my husband was not comfortable with the idea. He was more anxious about the birth than me, as this was his first baby. After going back and forth with me explaining why I wanted an experience different than my first birth, we compromised. I agreed to a hospital birth only if we could hire a doula to support us. I knew the benefits of hiring a doula and felt we needed the extra support.

Our doula, Jade, was amazing. She was actually an old school friend, which made her incredibly easy to talk to and trust. I appreciated her honesty, and valued her experience and knowledge. I also knew she would support us no matter what our decisions were. My husband and I had the opportunity to discuss our fears and Jade helped him prepare as a birth partner. I told her about my first birth experience, which I considered negative, and she was the first person I reached out to when my doctor completely violated my trust late in pregnancy.

At thirty-nine weeks, my obstetrician did a membrane sweep without my consent during a routine internal exam to check dilation. It was not effective at starting labor, which is no surprise. The traumatizing experience spiked my stress hormones enough to discourage it from starting! Labor did begin spontaneously six days past my daughter's estimated birth date after some time of grief and reflection.

My contractions began at 6 p.m. and I tried to remain comfortable as the surges started to become more intense. Our doula arrived shortly after 9 p.m. She asked me a few questions and then gently suggested I get out of bed. This was wonderful and eased some of the intensity I was feeling in my lower back. I was definitely experiencing back labor, which happens to one in four birthing people. I spent the next three hours at home going from the kitchen to the bathroom and into the shower—pacing all over. I learned a range of different positions for labor during pregnancy but honestly, the best feeling was standing. My body was my guide as I leaned over the kitchen counter while my husband and Jade took turns applying counter-pressure to my lower back.

My doula reminded me to eat and drink to keep my energy levels up and regularly brought a straw to my lips. I created privacy when I needed it by taking a shower. While there, I visualized my baby moving downward into my pelvis, just as the water from the shower flowed down my body. I also sat on the toilet, aka the "dilation station," for a while because that eased the intensity of my surges and opened up my pelvis in a different way.

Jade gave me prompts during and between contractions, which I appreciated. At one point she said, "Breathe your baby down," which I repeated to myself throughout the rest of labor. Near midnight, my husband suggested we leave for the hospital a few times. There was a snow storm and we knew it would take longer than usual to get there.

I put my husband off for a while saying, "Just a few more, just a few more," because while the contractions were intense, I wasn't finding them painful. I was annoyed by his suggestions to leave because I didn't feel ready. I had received Pitocin during my first labor and these contractions felt much more manageable in comparison. I had no idea how dilated I was but there was one thing I did know—I did not want to go to the hospital too soon! One of the ways I intended to avoid unnecessary interventions was to remain comfortable at home for as long as possible.

We left for the hospital and it took almost an hour to get there—double what it usually took. There was so much snow and we got stuck behind multiple snow plows. It was the most uncomfortable car ride of my life and later Jade told me she thought I was definitely in transition on the way— she thought I would give birth in her car!

When we got to the hospital, I was assessed and delighted to be 9 cm with "bulging waters," as the staff told me. I could not believe it because again, the contractions were nowhere near as painful as those brought on by the Pitocin I'd had last time. The nurses said I couldn't go into the hospital's labor pool because I was too close to having my baby. I was both disappointed and annoyed, but I was still able to take a shower, walk the halls and be upright—which were important to me.

I consented to intermittent fetal monitoring versus continuous but found even sitting on the bed to do this was very uncomfortable. There were no birth balls available for use at the time in 2012. I also found the staff wanted to keep checking on me, which I understood, but I felt an immense sense of pressure from them. My husband tried to act as my gatekeeper, coming into the shower saying, "They want to check you again," and I would emerge later when I was ready. I was trying to remain "in the zone" as much as I could but found it difficult. I did my best to relax, although I think the transfer from my home to the hospital significantly increased my anxiety. It also did not help that my non-consensual membrane sweep had happened in that hospital. I was paranoid that my boundary-crossing doctor would turn up at my birth for some reason. I never wanted to see him again.

During my labor both the on-call doctor and nurses looked at my bump and said, "Oh wow! You're definitely having a big baby!" *Un.help.ful.* The worst part? *When dilation stalled.* I spent four hours at 9 cm dilated with contractions coming fast and heavy. During the entire four hours I was never permitted into the pool. I got through them one at a time and tried not to focus on how much longer it would be until I met our baby.

My husband and doula took turns rubbing my lower back, cheering me on, telling me how well I was doing and most importantly, they kept me motivated when I started to get discouraged. There were times when I felt like my baby was not working with my body. I was able to voice this without shame or guilt to both of them. Jade reminded me of how strong I was and that I would meet my baby soon.

Deep down, I knew I needed something to get labor moving. I consented to the artificial rupture of my membranes. It was completely painless, however, there was meconium. My baby had made her first bowel movement while still in my womb, which can be a sign of fetal distress. I was told by the doctor and nurses that the pediatric team would need to come into the room and that my baby would need to be assessed to ensure she did not aspirate any meconium. Within moments of my waters being released (the doctor had not even left the room), I had the incredibly overwhelming sensation that I needed to push! I became very vocal and although I wanted to birth on all fours, kneeling or on my side, I was encouraged to get on my back.

The medical staff encouraged me to do coached pushing, but I did my own thing. This baby was coming and fast! She wanted to be born now and there was no way I could hold back. For a larger baby weighing in at 9 lbs 12 oz, she was out in three pushes. I remember right before that final push I felt so damn tired. My husband whispered words of encouragement into my ear that gave me the last bit of strength I needed to meet our daughter.

I was delighted when she was placed onto my chest briefly before being taken away for assessment.

My daughter was the only baby who was taken from my arms shortly after birth and I hated every second of it. I understood the need for her to be assessed and they did remove some meconium from her little tummy.

Thankfully, she had not aspirated any of it and she required no further monitoring. I would have rather had this process carried out while my baby was on my chest or next to me. Thankfully, she was returned to me within minutes so I could kiss, cuddle and smell her sweet baby scent. My doula congratulated our family and took some amazing pictures. She helped me establish breastfeeding for the first time and made sure all of us were comfortable before she left.

I felt so proud and strong after I'd had a chance to settle in with our daughter. There were times when I had doubted my ability and I was the queen of trying to compare this labor to my first labor. The fear of the unknown was my biggest hurdle and I had cleared it. My first baby was 6 lbs and this girl was almost ten! The nurses kept telling me I had a baby and a half, which made me laugh. The birth was much more positive than my first and I did it without pain relief, just as I had hoped. Breastfeeding was going well and I melted at the sight of my husband holding our daughter for the first time. Although she was born at almost 10 lbs, that did not stop everyone from commenting on how tiny she was!

While this birth experience was much, much more positive than my first, it was also my last birth in a hospital. What I learned is that personally, laboring in a hospital simply is not for me, if I can help it. The medicalized model of care with bright lights, loud beeps, more people in my birth space, medical equipment everywhere and the constant pressure from the medical staff to "move things along," was not helpful for my labor progression.

Everyone is going to be impacted by a clinical setting differently, however, I do not think it was a coincidence that my labor was going so smoothly at home and then BAM! I got to the hospital and all progression stalled for hours. How did my husband feel about everything? A few weeks postpartum he said, "I won't ever ask you to give birth in a hospital again." I think every expecting parent should have the opportunity to choose where they feel the most comfortable, safe and supported giving birth.

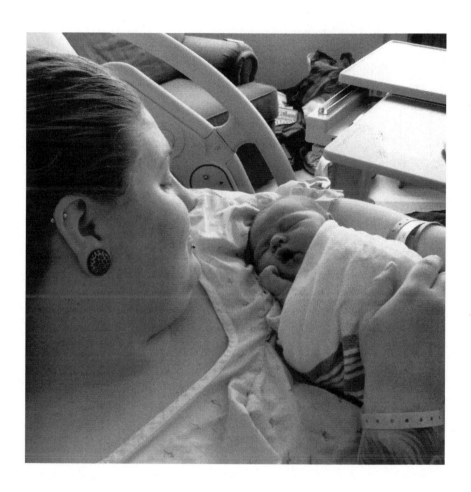

Michelle, United States:

My third pregnancy was by far my most challenging, with my body developing some symptoms of autoimmune health issues at six months of pregnancy. I was physically and emotionally drained and my mental health had taken a serious hit. My poor husband watched as my usual vibrant self crumbled under these new health concerns—thankfully, none of which were related to or impacting my pregnancy.

The path through my challenging pregnancy was paved by the excitement of meeting my baby and the love of family and friends. My husband and I wanted a home birth but sadly, with my health issues and a reduction in work hours as a result, we simply could not afford a midwife. Our insurance did not cover the cost of a private midwife and I was certain of one thing: I wanted to avoid giving birth in a hospital if possible. My last pregnancy ended with some unnecessary birth trauma and I struggled to feel safe and comfortable with the idea of birthing there again. After much research and discussion with friends who had chosen similar, we opted to give birth at home via freebirth.

My friend, who was also a trained birth doula, was happy enough to support us and we understood she was not a medical professional. We met with her regularly and she helped soothe some of my heightened anxiety levels. I also met with my obstetrician who knew of our plans and said that I was welcome to go to the hospital at any point and she would personally meet me to help with my baby's birth.

My baby's estimated birth date was the end of March and I repeatedly told my body that I trusted it to birth as it had twice before. I practiced a lot of meditation, especially when I found it challenging to sleep at night. I told my baby that I was ready to meet them whenever they were ready. Throughout my entire pregnancy I told friends that I wanted to follow my body's lead once labor began... and did I ever.

On April 9th, I still had no big indicators that labor was near. I had a passing thought that afternoon—*maybe things will start soon*, but it faded away just as quickly as it had entered my mind. Once I returned home from visiting my parents, I spent hours sitting on my birth ball. I went to bed that night just like all the ones previous, not feeling attached to labor starting or not. I trusted things to unfold however they were meant to. I was awakend at 4 a.m. by some intense twinges that felt very low in my pelvis. I changed positions a few times thinking that might help—no. I used the toilet thinking that might help—not a chance. These cannot be contractions, can they? They were so deep in my pelvis and not higher up in my uterus like in my previous births. I lay in bed and had a few more that were very strong—this must be it! I woke my husband, who started the birth pool set up.

Twenty minutes and at least three surges later, my husband asked if he should call our doula. I told him, "No! This could take hours!" but something immediately became different. The surges became more intense and were one on top of the other. I got a few bits and pieces ready for my birth space but yikes... what was happening? It felt like I was in transition but how could I be? I had only been in labor for thirty minutes.

I labored in the kitchen, often standing and leaning against the counter to support myself. I ordered my husband to ring our doula. I told her I needed her NOW! My husband hurried around trying to ensure the pool was filling while also trying to comfort me as I became louder. The surges were one right after the other and I felt like I had no opportunity to comprehend what was happening. I thought to myself, *this is either going to be the most painful labor ever or I'm in transition.*

I stood against my kitchen counter visualizing the surges like waves on a beach. Each one would swell, bring my baby closer to me and retreat again. Although they were very intense, I knew deep in my heart that the contractions were not something I had to fear. My body was obviously doing exactly what it needed to do in order to bring my baby down. I focused on my breath and my baby getting deeper into my pelvis. Within minutes of this, my waters released with a big gush and covered the kitchen floor. *I'm not losing my mind, baby is near.* The next two surges were the most intense as I simultaneously felt huge rectal pressure and movement in my pelvis. I knew I needed to get into the birth pool.

Those ten steps felt like ten miles but once I had got into the partially-filled pool, it was heaven. My husband followed as I got in and supported me as I rested my upper body against the side of the inflated pool. After my next surge, I reached down and said, "I can feel the baby's head!" I think this statement could still be the biggest shock of my husband's life. I had been in labor for just over an hour and there was only our family in the house—our doula had not made it yet. My hand rested on my baby's head and I remember thinking how small it felt. I was mindful about slowing down this stage of labor so my perineum could naturally stretch to reduce the chance of tearing.

One more surge and my baby was completely out. I did not have to actively push, as my body did all the work on its own—called the fetal ejection reflex. I brought our baby up to my chest, rubbed their back and felt my hands covered in vernix. I was so enamored while looking at my baby that I completely forgot to check the sex. I had a look only when my eleven-year-old son stepped into the room and asked what we had. I had given birth to a beautiful baby boy!

Our doula arrived forty-five minutes later when I was still in the pool bonding and feeding our baby boy, William. We glanced at the clock shortly following his birth and it was just after 5 a.m. I had been in labor from start to finish for only an hour and fifteen minutes!

William is now six and his intense personality is certainly in line with his very quick and overwhelming birth. Precipitous labors are defined as those lasting under three hours. They can feel overwhelming, stressful, shocking and even traumatizing for some. For us, I felt like this was the way our experience was meant to be and it was incredibly empowering and positive. I had hoped for an instinctual experience and that is exactly what my body brought me.

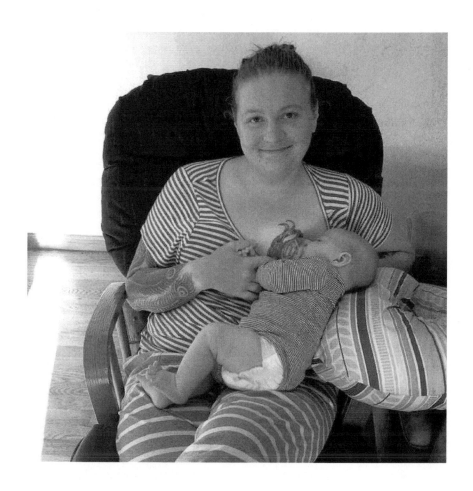

Michelle, Ireland:

It was December 2017 and my baby's estimated birth date had come and gone on the 18th. As forty weeks passed, I grew more impatient but also more hopeful that my baby would hopefully not be born on Christmas Eve or Christmas Day.

My baby did not arrive over the holidays and I found myself in my wonderful online "due date" group telling the other expecting parents that I was feeling emotionally and physically *done*. I was ready to meet my baby and I had a heart-to-heart with them, reassuring them that I was ready for labor whenever they were. I did not know it at the time, but hours later labor would begin.

At 8:30 that night I experienced a couple of tightening sensations very low in my pelvis, versus in the abdominal area. *Are these contractions?* I noted them and went about my evening putting kids to bed and preparing for a shower. Just before going in, I saw that I had begun to lose my mucus plug. I sent a message to my midwife and told my husband, "Tonight could be the night!" I showered and came out to see my husband and teenage son cleaning. They knew me well enough to know that giving birth in an untidy home would irritate me. We started a family board game as I sat on my exercise ball. I found myself both distracted and irritated. The "tightening sensations" were now clearly contractions, which I began to time via an app on my phone. They started to become more frequent and were manageable.

After the board game, my husband and I stayed up watching television and relaxing. The contractions started to slow at 11 p.m. so I suggested maybe a little intimacy would pick things up again. It did not so we decided to prioritize sleep—you never know how long labor will be. At 3 a.m., I was woken by contractions that were more intense and regular. I went downstairs and used both my CUB stool and birth ball to position myself as I watched more television and had a snack. The pool was being filled and my surges were approximately seven minutes apart, ranging from mild to moderate. At 6 a.m., my husband and I decided to cover the birth pool to help keep it warm and try to sleep again.

Surprisingly, my older children slept until 8 a.m. My contractions had slowed to thirteen to twenty minutes apart but when they did come, they were definitely more moderate. I wondered if my children being awake would decrease my oxytocin levels and thus slow my labor. I texted my midwife and promised to keep her updated. I felt certain my contractions would slow down or stop completely as the sun came up. From 8-9 a.m. we did our normal routine—ate breakfast and the kids quietly started playing with the toys they had got for Christmas. I told my husband things would probably not pick up so he could run to the shop and I would be fine at home... and oh, was I wrong!

Within thirty minutes of saying that, and just before he was about to leave, it felt like someone had flipped a switch. Suddenly my manageable contractions became challenging and I could not talk through them—hello active labor! I hunched over and breathed through them as they came every three to five minutes. My three older children being in the house suddenly became incredibly annoying. I quickly became irritated, especially with my husband. "I WANT THE KIDS OUT OF THE HOUSE NOW!"

My husband and I packed up the three kids with snacks, spare clothes and the "Nana and Grandad birth bag" that I had previously packed. The surges were now taking my breath away and making me cranky. My husband frantically tried to de-ice the car and broke the scraper in the process. He left with the kids, bringing them to my in-laws' house just five minutes away. (He later told me he was so afraid he was going to miss the birth while he was gone.) My husband was away and I texted my midwife three words—"I need you." It's honestly all I could think of and physically text. The surges came on fast and intense. Being alone for those fifteen minutes felt like an *eternity.* I felt much more emotionally overwhelmed by the surges when I was alone. I tried different labor positions, but nothing felt comfortable. I knew I had to get downstairs to the dining room where the birth pool was. I slowly made my way down between contractions as I tried to relax, although I was not very successful at that point.

The warmth of the birth pool was wonderful. I still felt deeply, deeply alone and couldn't wait for either the midwives or my husband to return. The midwives arrived first and let themselves in. My husband arrived a minute or two later. My vitals were taken and baby's heartbeat was checked— all was well. At this point I started to cry. I believe my body needed the endorphin release. When the kids were gone and I was surrounded by my support team, I suddenly realized and had to admit this was happening. I was in labor. This was going to be hard work and I had to lean into it to bring this new soul into the world.

I spent the next hour in the birth pool doing my deep breathing and visualization with hypnobirthing tracks playing in the background. They helped me focus on my breath and took my attention away from the intensity of my surges. The most comfortable laboring position was kneeling, but not on all fours. I kept looking at the vision board I had made and stuck to the wall. I read the positive birth affirmations and looked at the pictures of my three older children that I had intentionally chosen. Their smiling faces helped me get through the toughest parts. My husband was also amazing. He was on point with water, snacks and most importantly—he stayed near me. That was something I really craved during this labor more so than previous ones. He rubbed my shoulders, back and hips as needed intuitively. I felt like we were completely in-tune with each other. He wiped a cool cloth along my brow and helped me change positions as needed.

At one point I wanted to get out of the pool and into the bathroom. As I used the toilet, I heard a big *POP!* and my waters released. My midwife came in and asked if I thought my waters had gone. I told her more than once that I didn't know. It is clear to me now that I wasn't using my "thinking brain" but had started to rely on my primitive brain. This one question required more energy and attention to answer than I was willing to give. (I look back at this moment and chuckle because it was so obvious that yes, my amniotic sac had burst!) I felt really comfortable sitting on the toilet, but my midwife urged me to get back into the pool. She clearly knew I was closer to birth than I did. I slowly made my way back to the pool, not knowing if it would be minutes or hours until my baby arrived.

During the next contraction, I felt indescribable bulging in my perineum. *Wait. Wait. Wait!* I thought to myself, *How is this possible? I haven't been actively pushing!* This is the beauty of the human body. Your body and your baby know when it is time. My uterine muscles had been pushing my baby down without me consciously doing so. The next contraction brought my baby's head to my vaginal opening. I was so overwhelmed because again, I had not been actively pushing. I said, "Help me, help me, help me!" because of the pure overwhelm when I realized my baby would be emerging right at that moment.

Truth be told, just minutes earlier I thought I had hours to go before this baby would be born. The two midwives quickly came to my side and instructed me on how to breathe to slow the crowning process. I am so happy they were there! Two seconds later and my baby's head emerged... and there it rested for a while. I told my husband to get my phone and there are several pictures of me with our baby's head just outside of my body. I kept my hand on my baby's head as this happened...

My baby's head turned not once, not twice, but three times after it had emerged with my hand gently resting on it. I also felt the baby's body turn while still inside me several times. This was amazing. Intellectually, I knew the baby's body would make an internal rotation before fully emerging, but to be so present during birth as to feel it was something new to me. I felt everything!

One small push later and the rest of my baby's body emerged at 11:03 a.m. on December 27th. My baby's eyes were wide open and the umbilical cord rested across the back of the neck. I gently released it, lifted the baby to my chest and sat back as a towel was draped over us both. I looked and we had a baby boy!

I think back to this experience and it was absolutely everything I wanted from a home birth. I trusted my body and I had a supportive duo of midwives who believed in my ability to birth my baby too. My husband stepped up to be the amazing support person I needed. I have never felt more in love with him than I did then. We welcomed our baby calmly and peacefully, just as we had hoped.

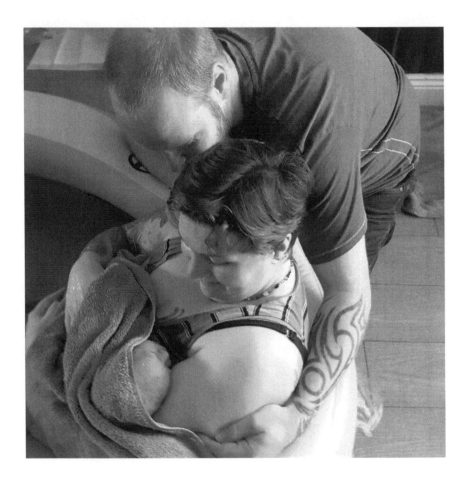

Michelle, Ireland:

I found myself at the end of my fifth pregnancy feeling a desire to cherish the experience. I think many people feel this way, especially during their last pregnancy. As much as I wanted to continue holding onto my pregnancy, I wanted to hold my baby in my arms more. These feelings started to grow more intense on July 14th, two days past my baby's estimated birth date, and I started communicating with my little one. "Okay, I'm done with this pregnancy business. It's time to meet, babe!"

Within twelve hours of this heart-to-heart and following a decent night's sleep, I began to lose my mucus plug at 9 a.m. on July 15th. I became excited, knowing that for me this was a good sign that labor was at least nearer. I spent the morning cleaning the last few bits for my planned home birth and relaxing. I prefer to labor at night so I had no desire to do anything to promote daytime labor. I ate, I drank, I watched a romcom, I did some movements upright on my birth ball and at 2 p.m. attempted to take a nap with my toddler. I listened to my hypnobirthing tracks as I tried to sleep; by now some light surges had started. They were low, very manageable and sporadic—being anywhere from fifteen to forty-five minutes apart.

I still felt like I did not want to promote labor and the surges stopped completely at 6 p.m. My family and I continued life as normally as we could—we had dinner, I showered and the kids played outside. Just before bed time, we removed the table and chairs from the dining room and brought out the birth pool and foam mats—all of which the kids found incredibly amusing.

Once our youngest three children were in bed, my husband and I took a very short walk after 10 p.m. and sure enough, the surges started up again just as I had predicted they would. They immediately began being five to seven minutes apart and forty-five to sixty seconds long. I knew this change was because I felt better able to relax. My husband and sixteen-year-old son began filling the birth pool while I continued listening to my hypnobirthing tracks. I felt safe and comfortable adding sound to my exhales, which promoted the softening of my jaw and even deeper relaxation. I retreated upstairs at midnight to my dark bedroom where I lay on my side in bed, hoping I might catch a few minutes' sleep. I rang Ann, my midwife, and asked her to join us, knowing she had a two-hour drive ahead of her.

Shortly after, my husband came upstairs visibly upset and tearful, stating we had a serious problem. The birth pool, which we had done a trial run with, had a leak! This was the same birth pool I had used two times previously and we had no patch kit! Water had slowly saturated the floor from a puncture in the bottom of the pool. Clearly this was not how I had envisioned my birth. My surges immediately became more intense, no doubt a response to the stress hormones which I am certain my body started pumping out in response to this news.

Thankfully I remembered my hypnobirthing techniques and it was still early enough for me to ring someone for help. I jumped into problem-solver mode. A doula friend had a birth pool and liner I could use, but she was a forty-minute drive away. I called another friend, Marta, and she agreed to collect it for me, thankfully. The idea of my husband having to leave me at home for that length of time filled me with dread, so I was relieved we had help.

12:30 a.m.: Midwife on the way? Check. Birth pool situation being remedied? Check. My birth photographer notified? Check.

My husband and son emptied the punctured pool and filled some large plastic storage containers with the warm water. Problem-solving at its finest. This way the water could simply be transferred into the new pool, assuming it arrived before baby did.

Labor became increasingly challenging. I was waiting on everyone to get to the house as the surges became more and more intense. I had hoped the surges would space out but it was not meant to be. My heart was set on a waterbirth so the idea of dealing with the intensity of labor without the soothing warmth and buoyancy filled me with dread. There were times when I panicked, but I did my best to listen to my hypnobirthing tracks, practice the breathing techniques and visualize my body opening and releasing. As a birth doula, I was well aware of all the different labor positions, but I chose to sit in a nursing chair rocking my way through the surges. Meanwhile, my husband held my hand, gently massaged my arm and legs and tried to organize things between the surges while we waited for people to start arriving.

Every time he left my side, even if it was to help me directly, I awaited his return with every single fiber in my body. I needed to feel his skin on mine and the love he had for me. I could feel my fear building and I used every hypnobirthing technique I knew to help bring me back down to a place of more calm. It was a cycle of positive self-talk, breathing and trusting that my birth would unfold in whatever way it was meant to. I

MICHELLE MAYEFSKE

chose to focus on the things I could control, which was my response to the situation and bringing my attention back to the fact that I would be meeting my baby very soon!

Marta arrived with the pool at 2 a.m. and my surges were now approximately three minutes apart. I felt a mixture of relief and impatience when she arrived. Marta suddenly became my unplanned hand-holding and body-soothing companion through the increasingly stronger surges. My husband and son focused on the pool and I was adamant that I *needed* someone by my side at all times. The surges kept moving lower, a throbbing in my upper thighs became overwhelming and I got increasingly more vocal as my discomfort increased.

My midwife arrived within ten minutes and the pure relief of her arrival was amazing. I had a chance to express my frustrations—I wanted that damn pool filled, I felt uncomfortable in the rocking chair but also did not want to move and I was very adamant that I now needed two people near me.

I told Ann on multiple occasions not to leave my side. Marta and Ann held my hands, put counter pressure on my legs to ease the throbbing, offered me water, put a cool cloth on my forehead and Ann coached me through the surges that had reached a serious peak. (Ann later told me my hypnobirthing was clearly helping because my hands were completely limp, even during my surges. I was not tensing up or squeezing. This made me so happy to hear.) Ann's words comforted me when my breathing became more frantic and I felt myself starting to spin to a place of momentary panic. I also called my husband over, requesting his presence when the surges felt particularly challenging. He really was being pulled in all directions!

At one stage I knew I needed to release the idea of birthing in the birth pool, even if it was currently being filled. I told Ann I could feel the baby moving down but that I felt like I was holding back because I desperately wanted to be in the pool. Ann reminded me that this was my last pregnancy and that I could enjoy this birth. Wrapping my head around that was so challenging. I believe my initial internal dialogue said *fuck off*, but then I reminded myself that Ann was right—I had the ability to enjoy the process.

I asked about the pool at least ten times while simultaneously trying not to obsess or focus on it too much. I wanted to desperately ask Ann how much longer I had to go, and while I knew she could guess based on her expertise, I also feared she could be wrong. (Ann told me later that she could tell I was fully dilated already upon her arrival). I was beginning to tremble. I told Ann I was scared; I was sweating buckets and I felt like I could not go on—all signs birth was near!

As 3 a.m. approached, my headphones were still in with tracks playing, although even the max bluetooth volume was annoyingly too low to fully block out the commotion around me. I knew I was in transition and I asked Marta and my husband to swap places. Burco boilers and pans on the stove were relentlessly heating water and I needed Marta to take over that task so he could be near me in the rocking chair. I managed to say that I was getting in that pool now, no matter how full or warm it was. My intuition told me I would completely open and soften my pelvic floor once I got into the water, something I struggled with while in the chair. Ann helped me over and I had a surge while standing supported by her. It was much easier to manage versus being seated and I regretted not trying to stand earlier!

As I climbed into the water, I felt it was a tad too warm and I requested cold water to even it out. The amazing otherworldly relief of that pool has to be one of the most magical moments of my life. I instantly knew my baby would come any minute. My husband was setting up the video camera as I told him, "If you want to meet your baby, you better get over here now!"

I knew the position would be intense, but I knelt with my legs wide apart while supporting my upper body on the inflatable seat built into the pool. My husband was on my left and Ann on my right. I needed them both as I could feel the heaviness of my baby's head already in my pelvis. My husband poured warm water down my back as I waited for the next surge to come. This felt heavenly and I remember smiling on the inside and outside because I knew my baby was moments away. I had made it this far.

It took four surges in the pool and my baby's head and body were born at 3:06 a.m. I was only in the pool for ten minutes total. I honestly felt complete euphoria and shock. I got through labor, my baby was born in water as I had hoped and *I did it* even when things became challenging. I gently lifted our baby from beneath the water, seeing that my prediction was right and we had a little girl. Within the first minute of birth I was laughing, smiling, crying, kissing and talking to our baby. The first things I noticed were her long nails, the vernix on her skin and her full head of hair. I excitedly said to my husband, "Isn't she beautiful!" as Ann commented that she looked big. Then I said she *felt* big.

My two children, ages eight and five, were unbeknownst to me waiting in our front hallway. The looks on their faces when they saw me and their baby sister in the pool were priceless.

The rest of our story involves clean up, passing the placenta, doing umbilical cord burning, family photos, baby's fetal check and weight (10 lbs, 13 oz. with no stitches needed) and loads of chat about the birth. I said to Marta, "I bet you didn't think you would be staying for my entire birth tonight!" and we all laughed together at the swiftness of what had just happened. My daughter's birth was a step away from the ultra-calm birth I had imagined, however, it was incredibly positive and I think baby Iris was born exactly how she was meant to be.

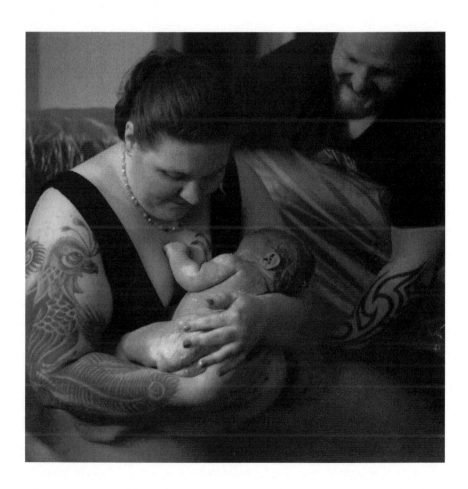

Anonymous:

It was a wonderful surprise to find out that we were expecting our first baby in the midst of a global pandemic. The entire world seemed to have gone mad, but we were able to insulate ourselves in our little bubble of delight at home. Little did we know that our baby would be born during this pandemic and just how much that would impact our decisions and experiences.

I had a hospital appointment at twelve weeks where my BMI came up in three conversations with three separate people. I was immediately categorized as a high-risk patient and a consultant who barely spoke to me prescribed me aspirin and a test for gestational diabetes. This was all done before she even looked at me.

This is not how I would define care—it was a conveyor belt system. After this experience, I made the decision to pursue private obstetric care. This would help us to achieve continuity of care and enable me to avoid attending the hospital until birth. I wanted to know the person who would assist with the birth of my baby. It would also insulate us from as much of the ongoing pandemic as possible.

I located a clinic and an obstetrician who operated in my chosen hospital. The consultant I chose was wonderful and had no focus on my BMI. We focused on conversations around health—eating lots of fresh food for good nutrition, to grow a healthy baby and set myself up for recovery. There was never a conversation about my size, as it should be. Informed consent was huge in this clinic. Before each exam or scan I was asked the question, "Is it okay if I have a feel of your tummy? Would it be okay to do a scan and look at baby today?" Every choice was placed on me.

The birth I imagined was in a hospital, a natural labor and delivery, with minimal pain medication, soothing music and a swift discharge home. My little baby would latch on and breastfeed happily and we could doze away in newborn bliss. The only thing I wanted to avoid was a cesarean, however, there is nothing like pregnancy, birth and motherhood to make you consider all options.

The pregnancy was relatively straightforward with a scatter of minor ailments throughout, the most distressing of which was severe carpal tunnel syndrome affecting both hands from thirty-one weeks onwards. Baby was growing healthy, but it was getting increasingly more painful for me. I could not lift a cup by the time I went into the clinic for my thirty-eight-week checkup. It was agony and the prescribed paracetamol did little to ease the pain. Coupled with pregnancy-induced insomnia, I was awake for at least twenty-two hours of every day to really indulge in the pain!

To my delight both the midwife and the consultant could clearly see things had progressed past reasonable and we were able to sit down and discuss a birth plan. The first option put to me was an induction. From my examination we knew that baby was still sitting very high in my pelvis and had not yet engaged. I was not showing any signs of being favorable for induction. We discussed honestly how the induction process might look for my individual circumstance. It could potentially be a lengthy process, even a couple of days. They could not guarantee anything, and I asked to be informed of the possible outcomes.

An induction for a first-time mother with my presentation had a relatively high chance of ending in an assisted delivery or potentially an emergency cesarean. With the current hospital restrictions, my partner would not be by my side until I was in active labor and transferred to the labor ward. I was informed this would be when I was 4 cm dilated. The thought of going through multiple internal exams, hours of frustration and potentially pain, without the support of my birth partner was very upsetting. I took the plunge and asked the question, "What about a c-section?"

My doctor explained the risks first. It is a major abdominal surgery, there is a risk of damage to the bladder and bowel of the mother. Babies born via cesarean are more likely to need assistance breathing and clearing mucus, as they have not gone through the natural birth process. I was also told a cesarean could make initiating breastfeeding more challenging. I wanted to know how soon I could be discharged and he said I would be discharged after two days, provided recovery was smooth.

The third option was obviously to wait for labor to begin on its own. I was exhausted and in agony, which was taking its toll on my health. My blood pressure was creeping up, my anxiety was increasing and my headspace was tipping the scale into a little too negative. This was the option I was able to rule out first. I spent a long time with the consultant that day asking different questions and weighing up the different options. As always, he was very factual, and everything was my choice. He leaned neither way.

I told him to book the cesarean. There were three reasons.
- I would have my partner there all the way.

- I would have a known amount of time in hospital.
- I was so exhausted, induction was terrifying for me.

So, I went home, I repacked my bags and Tuesday rolled around quickly. We arrived at the hospital at 7 a.m., and I went off for my pre-op checks. I had been harvesting colostrum from thirty-six weeks, so I had 80 ml of frozen breast milk to send to the fridge for my baby's first feed. It was important to me that she would get what nature intended as her first meal.

I met my midwife who sat with me and we chatted about the upcoming holiday, Christmas. I walked down to theater with the midwife and my birth partner at 11 a.m. After my spinal block was placed, my partner took a seat by my left shoulder and the drapes went up. My consultant came in and asked me was I ready to meet my baby—of course I was!

At 11:28 a.m., there was a gush of water and a little gurgle of a new baby as the consultant lifted the baby over the drapes and said, "Meet your baby girl!" My partner was able to capture this moment in a photo that I will forever cherish. I was over the moon.

My baby fell into the known risks for babies born via cesarean, as she struggled to breath straight away. The pediatrician was looking after her and the decision was made to take her to the special care unit for some assistance. I was upset, although I did know this might happen. I sent my partner to be with her while the surgery was finished. Afterwards, the consultant came around to congratulate me and said all had gone well and he would see me back on the ward.

Once I was back in the postnatal ward, I was looking for my baby. I wanted her and I wanted her *now*. She was only up the hall but still needed assistance for her breathing and some monitoring. I was stuck in bed, numb from the spinal block. I was told that once I was mobile again, I could sit with her for as long as I wanted in the special care unit.

Just six hours after my spinal was placed, I was up and walking the halls to prove a point—I could do this and I was going to be with my baby! The older midwives told me to take it easy and go back to bed, but the midwife I trusted told me, "Motion is lotion." The more you move, the better you will feel—while obviously being careful not to overdo it. I hobbled up to special care to meet my sweet girl. From there on I sat in a comfy chair in special care only returning to my room when I had to. I felt a huge urge to stay with her.

In total, my girl spent thirty-six hours in the special care unit to stabilize her breathing and blood sugars. Breastfeeding was not off to the start I had imagined. She was so sleepy she just would not latch, even giving a bottle was proving hard work for this girl. She had taken the colostrum I had saved for her and I was now expressing to get milk into her anyway we could.

Fast forward another six weeks and my daughter was still a very sleepy baby. We had all the newborn checks, so this is just the way nature made her. My own recovery after the cesarean was very smooth. I had no complications whatsoever. My wound healed quickly and very well. I was originally concerned about this because I have an apron belly and the incision site was right there. Thankfully, it did not cause me any issues. Just four days after the cesarean, I felt better than I had before birth. At six weeks on, I barely felt I had surgery at all.

I felt grateful to my care providers for always keeping me informed and making me feel valued and safe throughout my pregnancy and birth. My birth and journey as a new mother was nothing like what I had imagined it to be, but it was still perfect.

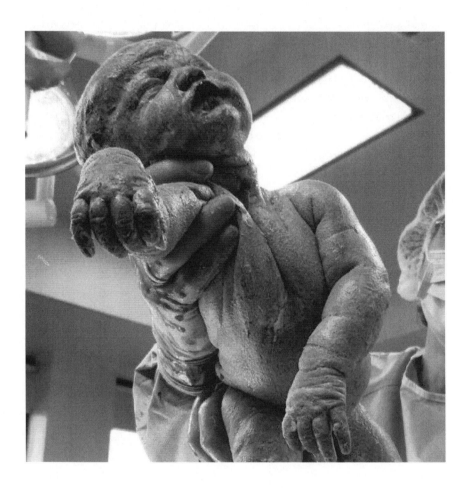

Chloe, Ireland:

** *Content warning for weight stigma in a medical setting.*

My pregnancy was fairly standard, with absolutely no complications. I escaped hyperemesis gravidarum, the severe pregnancy sickness my mother suffered with during all three of her pregnancies. She warned me before my booking appointment, having had three plus size pregnancies herself, that the maternity staff would comment a lot on my weight and BMI. She told me to speak up, not be afraid to tell them to stop and set boundaries. I nodded along as she spoke, just as I knew I would in the maternity unit.

I met my first midwife at my booking appointment. She was a fantastic lady who considered not only my BMI but my entire lifestyle as well. I was going to the gym four times a week and was healthy overall, so she suggested the midwives clinic. I was on a positive high as I went on to meet the doctor. He was not interested in me. He did not even say hello before he went straight into my medical file. "Okay, very high BMI, not good at all—no midwife clinic for you. It's recommended that someone your size take aspirin for the entire pregnancy, as you will probably get preeclampsia. I'm also prescribing calcium and vitamin D, as I doubt you get enough. You should go on a diet and you need a diabetes test at twenty-eight weeks, as big people usually get that." He left the room while my jaw was still on the ground. That was the end of my positive high.

I passed my glucose tolerance test but was told I needed to repeat it at thirty-two weeks, as the baby was measuring big and I had extra amniotic fluid. From thirty weeks onward the baby was measuring big, but I was not surprised. My mum and aunt also had big babies with zero complications. My aunt delivered a boy at home unmedicated. My results from my second glucose test were normal; however, they considered having me take a third glucose tolerance test because they assumed me being fat meant I must have had gestational diabetes and not just that I had made a big baby.

At my last appointment at thirty-seven weeks I finally met a doctor who agreed—I was just making a big baby without any gestational diabetes diagnosis. He scheduled me for an induction the following Monday at thirty-eight weeks due to my baby's estimated size.

I was admitted Monday morning; however, my waters burst all over the doctor and midwife during my internal cervical check. I started labor at noon and joined my husband for walks in the car park. Hospital restrictions meant I was mostly unable to have my husband beside me during the worst of the contractions. I was finally 4 cm at 11:30 p.m. and moved to the labor ward where my husband could join me. I told myself I was open to the epidural and by midnight, did I want it. At 12:30 a.m., I had jumped to 8 cm so the midwives and the anesthesiologist rushed to get me the epidural in time. They were a wonderful team and I was able to get a bit of rest once it was placed. At 3:00 a.m., the midwives explained how to push and told me to practice a couple. Four sets of pushes and forty minutes later, I had an 8 lbs 15 oz baby boy in my arms! I held him and cried while the team continued to work away on me, without complaint. I only had a small tear on one side—*thank you perineal massage!* They let us stay over two hours, with my husband getting skin to skin and me learning how to breastfeed baby. Not once was my weight an issue that day. I labored on my own without complications.

I was so proud of myself and my postpartum healing went well. A person's weight does not predict how their pregnancy will go, even if some people say otherwise.

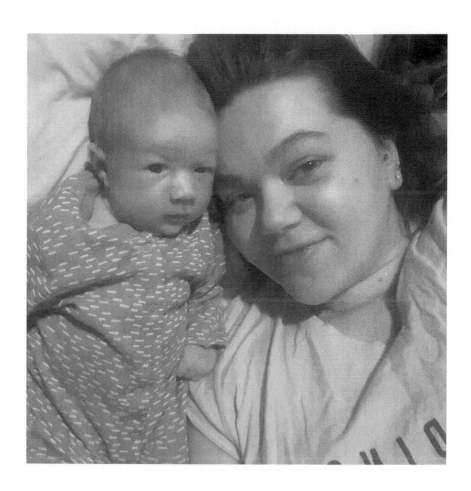

Marta Korpys, Ireland:

** *Weight stigma in a medical setting.*

I was so excited and happy throughout all of my pregnancy. I had some typical pregnancy symptoms—heartburn, swelling in my legs and carpal tunnel syndrome during my last month. I put on a lot of weight during my pregnancy, but this didn't bother me because I still had a lot of energy. I worked my entire pregnancy until I reached eight months. My husband, Krzysztof, and I were also busy doing work in our home—painting rooms and preparing for our baby's arrival.

Krzysztof and I visited our native Poland when I was five months pregnant. We booked a private scan so we could see our baby in 4D and learn the sex. I was lying there for the scan and the sonographer was incredibly rude. She said, "I can't see the face of your baby because you have too much fat on your belly."

I was looking forward to having some scan photos printed as a keepsake, but she didn't print any for us. The only positive thing about this experience was we learned we were having a baby girl.

I was happy with the maternity care I received when we returned to Ireland. The only information I had regarding pregnancy was based on stories from my friends living in Poland. I quickly learned that in Poland it is typical to have more antenatal visits than I was having in Ireland. There is also more routine testing in Poland. For example, everyone has a glucose tolerance test there. I also felt there was an overall cultural difference regarding pregnancy—in Poland your pregnancy is acknowledged from the date you receive your first positive pregnancy test. This is in contrast to Ireland, where, in my opinion, pregnancies are often not recognized until you reach twelve weeks.

My general practitioner saw me in early December and signed me off work because of swelling in my legs. They didn't test me for preeclampsia. During the third trimester I also began perineal massage to hopefully prevent tearing or needing an episiotomy during birth. I did this myself and Krzysztof helped as my bump got bigger.

My baby's estimated birth date was January 7th, and I had lost some of my mucus plug just before Christmas. My mom came to visit from Germany during that time and I thought it would be lovely for her to be with us if I gave birth—sadly, it was not meant to be.

At my thirty-nine-week appointment, my consultant asked if I would like a membrane sweep, and I consented. It was ineffective at starting labor so I was back in his office again at forty weeks. It was then he said I would be induced if I did not go into labor on my own by forty-two weeks.

On January 18th at 5 p.m., I started to feel some light cramping while relaxing in our sitting room. Like many first-time moms, I was not 100 percent sure I was in labor. Light contractions started coming every fifteen minutes until midnight. I took a shower and lie awake in bed as the cramps started happening more often. My waters broke at 4 a.m., but I was not sure if it really was my waters—the leaking was minimal and not a big gush. I rang the maternity unit at 5 a.m. and the contractions were now five minutes apart. The midwives told me not to go in until my waters broke. I remained home until there was a big gush of my amniotic fluid at 10 a.m. We packed and left for the maternity hospital, arriving at noon.

When we arrived, another big gush of my waters came while I was seated in the car, absolutely soaking me. I was wet and cold, laboring in the car on a January day. I decided to change in the car before going into hospital admissions—that was interesting! I received an internal exam once inside the hospital and was told I was 3 cm dilated. Krzysztof and I were sent to the antenatal ward where my labor continued. The contractions were now getting more and more intense.

Krzysztof was hungry at 2 p.m. and I told him to get something to eat because he is diabetic. I didn't want anything to eat because I had already vomited in admissions. Once my husband returned, we walked the hospital corridors for a while. A midwife did another internal exam and I was 6 cm dilated at 5 p.m.

I was moved to the labor ward where midwives offered me the use of pain relief. I decided to use gas and air, but I was only biting on it rather than inhaling how you are supposed to. I got on the floor to lean against the bed and changed into other positions to help relieve the intensity of the contractions. My blood pressure was being monitored and had been increasing since I was admitted to the hospital. The doctor gave me medication to help bring it down, but it was ineffective after two attempts. The doctor and midwives said they needed to do something about it, as high blood pressure wasn't good for me or my baby. They said the only other thing they could offer was an epidural, as a common side effect of its use is reducing blood pressure.

It was 10 p.m. and I was 8 cm dilated at this stage. I wondered why I really needed the epidural if I was so close to 10 cm. I had friends who were denied an epidural when they were this far along in labor, yet I was being told I needed it now. I was undecided on what to do. My worries were mostly about any complications from the epidural affecting me in the future. I talked with Krzysztof about everything and ultimately we decided to go ahead, hoping the epidural would stabilize my blood pressure. The midwives were great at going through how the epidural would work and helped me remain still while it was administered. I was disappointed when I got the epidural because I had wanted to go through labor without it; however, the hospital staff were right—it did bring my blood pressure down.

I was much calmer and felt relief immediately after the epidural was placed. I could not feel pain or much pressure, but I could feel some movement. I was lying there for an hour and then I started to feel the sensations of the contractions coming back to me. The midwives said, "That cannot be possible," but they believed me when I became more vocal! They did top up my epidural at midnight, and they encouraged me to lie down and continue resting. I was drifting in and out of sleep for an hour and at 1 a.m., I was 10 cm dilated.

The midwives began guiding me on when and how to push, by watching my contractions on the monitor. I found it hard to push because I could not feel where I was pushing—the sensation was gone. I did not feel like I was pushing very hard or doing an effective job, but the midwives said I was doing great.

Baby Cora arrived at 1:25 a.m. weighing 8 lbs 3 oz. She was placed straight onto my chest, where she looked up at me with one little eye open. I noticed straight away that she was so clean—no blood or vernix on her.

Krzysztof cut the umbilical cord and explained how amazing it was to see Cora crowning. As she was coming out, the plates of her skull that had molded during birth were moving back out to their normal position! Some of my friends had said things like, "Don't let him look—he will never want to have sex with you again," but I did not believe that. I was happy that Krzysztof got to watch our baby being born as he supported my leg.

Throughout all of labor, Kryzysztof was a wonderful support for me. As Cora breastfed, he mentioned how sore his legs were from standing for so many hours. He had been afraid to say something or sit down when I was going through the waves of my labor!

I enjoyed my tea and toast before going to the postnatal ward with my baby girl. We enjoyed incredible bonding through more lovely skin to skin and breastfeeding.

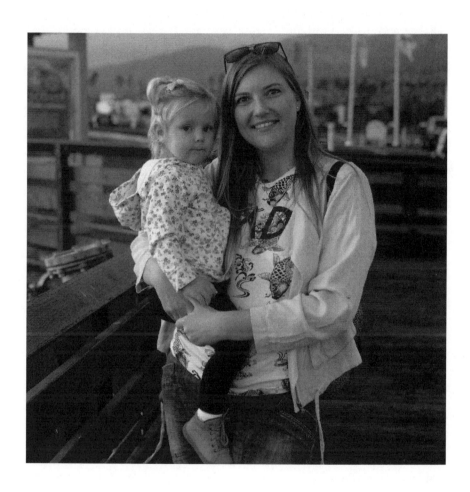

Mikaylea:

I was well into my third trimester with a very low-key pregnancy as I prepared for my home birth. On July 3rd, 2019 I had an appointment where I told my midwife that I didn't feel well. Everything felt foggy, tired and just... off. I knew something was wrong, but I did not know exactly what. My blood pressure that day was 178/110 so I needed to have my blood and urine tested. I was put on bed rest, given magnesium and put on a blood-pressure diet.

The next day, my midwife came by my house to see how I was; I felt no change. Protein was found in my urine by test strips and my blood pressure was still high even though I had been in bed all day. We headed to the hospital for emergency labs and to consult with an obstetrician. The walk-in lab was very limited and did not seem concerned, as it was the American holiday—the 4th of July. They said my labs should be back within a day or two.

The next day they called and said my blood work was borderline for preeclampsia but my urine test was not back yet. The obstetrician wanted me to rest and come into his office four days later to get blood pressure medication and indicated that my planned home birth should still be able to go ahead.

Another day passed and I still did not feel well at all. That afternoon I got a call from my midwife—my urine results came back from a few days prior and my protein levels were through the roof. She told me to go to the hospital immediately and she would meet me there. Once we arrived, the hospital retested my urine since it had been a few days—my protein levels had more than doubled at over 13,000! They wanted to induce me immediately. I was eighteen years old and thirty-six weeks and one day pregnant at the time. I was scared for me and my baby and I was crushed that I had to be in the hospital. My peaceful waterbirth vision was gone, but I still wanted to go through labor without using pain medication.

The nurse started me on Pitocin, increasing the dosage often. She asked how I was feeling when the dosage hit five. I told her I was doing okay, uncomfortable yet it was manageable. She told me, "I'm going to come in here and keep giving you more until you're in 10/10 pain and screaming for me to give you an epidural," then walked out.

I was shocked but ignored her statement. I could do this, I knew I could.

After a few hours, I was 4 cm dilated, making slow progress, but progress nonetheless. It continued to get challenging and intense. The only comfortable position I could be in was on the birth ball. We were having issues keeping track of my baby's heart rate on the monitor, which was so frustrating and disheartening. They made me get back into the bed multiple times which was very uncomfortable.

I got to 9 cm and felt like I might need to push. The nurse turned off my Pitocin and forced me to lay down with my legs closed, saying I needed to wait for the doctor because he had not even left his house yet. I had regressed to 5 cm dilated by the time he arrived. He told me I was not making any progress at all and that he was going to break my waters and turn the Pitocin back up. I told him no, that I would think about it. I felt like he wasn't treating me well or that he thought I wasn't competent, although I was. I don't know if he assumed I was a dumb teen mom or not, but it was frustrating.

I did eventually decide to have my waters broken, which I instantly regretted. The pain intensified immediately. I was in so much pain I just wanted to be done. I didn't think I could go on anymore. I wanted to get in the shower; however, because they couldn't get the monitors to work, they wouldn't permit me to unless I had an internal fetal monitor. I really didn't want one but consented because I needed the freedom to move. I got in the shower and cried to my mom. I told her I couldn't do it and that it hurt. She told me I could do it, that I was doing it and that it would end soon. I was completely exhausted at this point and could barely hold myself up, so I went back onto the bed and laid down. I tried to rest between the peaks of contractions but I was not getting much of a break between them.

This part is all a blur because of how tired I was. After a while, I felt like I needed to be on my hands and knees, so I rested my weight on the bed while bent over. It was so intense at this point—I thought I might break. A new doctor came in but I hardly noticed. He quietly watched me from the corner, came over, and gently asked if he could check me. I said yes. I did not even notice him checking me as another contraction hit.

"You're almost nine centimeters. You're almost done. You've got this," he told me.

Not long after I started to feel more and more like I needed to push. I pushed for quite a while on my hands and knees, but I was so swollen from the preeclampsia that I couldn't feel my legs or anything. I had gone purple from the blood pooling in my legs. I lay half on my side, still totally exhausted, so I could barely hold myself up. My sister held my leg in the air, my husband held my hand and my mom told me over and over that I could do it. My midwives encouraged me as the doctor was silent— hands-off watching... waiting...

My body pushed for what felt like hours, but in reality I don't know exactly how long it was. I remember asking if I was almost done and one of my midwives telling me, "Reach down, touch your baby. Her head is right there!"

I reached down and felt her head, not quite crowning but she would be soon. I sobbed with relief that I was finally almost done—my baby was almost here. I pushed with the next contraction, and I screamed, "It burns, it burns! Why does it burn?!"

I knew what the "ring of fire" was but it still caught me by surprise. My other midwife coached me to relax and blow through the next contraction. Just as I thought I would have to endure another contraction and push again, the doctor told me, "You can pick up your baby!"

Her head had been born and I did not even feel the rest of her body come out. I reached down and brought her to my chest. I sobbed and said over and over that I loved her and she was so beautiful. She was perfect— completely healthy and alert. She needed no assistance or NICU time, had no feeding problems and weighed in at 6 lbs 11 oz. It was not the birth I had envisioned but it was beautiful in its own right.

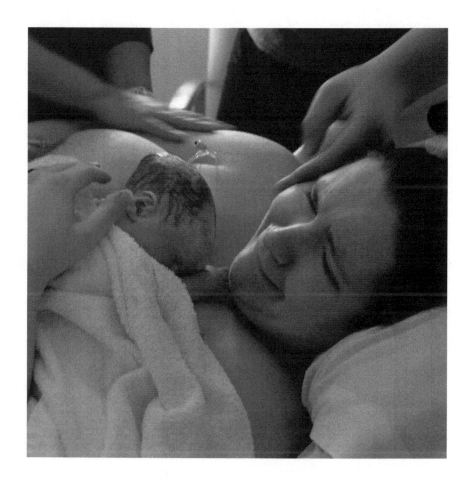

Laura McQuade, United States:

*** Content warning for weight stigma in a medical setting.*

I started my pregnancy as a "super plus size" person and from the very beginning, my experience was haunted by foretellings of doom. The first attending nurse I saw kept repeating that pregnancy at my size is "very risky" and that, "You have options—you're only eight weeks, and still young."
From that point no one was as blunt, but the implication was clear in every medical interaction: either my baby or I were not going to survive my pregnancy or birth.

They were so wrong! I had a picture-perfect pregnancy the whole way through. My baby developed beautifully and I was more at peace with my body than ever before. Because of the associated "risks" for someone my size, my doctor suggested an induction at thirty-seven weeks, and I consented. I was so eager to meet my little girl. It took three days for labor to progress far enough and I spent the whole time on fetal monitors. The medical staff were so sure something would go wrong—but it never did.

I had an epidural around midnight and at 10 a.m., after just an hour of pushing, we met baby Máire for the first time. I was surprised it had been an hour, as it felt like maybe fifteen minutes. Just over 7 lbs of beautiful baby rested on my chest and eagerly looked around the room. She smiled when she heard her Papa call her name and tried to lift her head right away.

I was done bleeding and back to 90 percent of my pre-pregnancy endurance by six weeks postpartum. My body grew and birthed my perfect baby girl with zero complications and that is the greatest gift the universe could give me.

Marianne, Ireland:

** Content warning for pregnancy loss.

My birth story is different from some—I fall into the category of one in four. I gave birth to my baby girl at full term when she was thirty-eight weeks, but sadly we did not get to keep her. Lily had died a few days before she was born.

In early June 2019, I noticed that my baby had not reacted to a loud bang and we went into hospital on a Saturday morning. I had a scan and we were told the worst words parents ever want to hear, "Guys, I'm so sorry. There's no heartbeat."

Lily was thirty-eight weeks exactly and I had my baby shower planned for later that day. Next came shock, anger and disbelief. We were given time to ourselves and the doctor came back and explained the process. I remember wanting to have her taken out of me straight away. The staff explained gently that it would be better for me to have a vaginal delivery so that there would not be any complications in future pregnancies.

I was so numb that I followed the advice they gave me. In the room where we had the ultrasound, they gave me drugs that would suppress pregnancy hormones and help me start labor. We were told to go home and come back on Monday for an induction. We went home, grieved and waited. Even though it was summer, we both were shivering when we got back to the house—in hindsight, it was shock and not the cold.

On the Monday, I was admitted to a ward that had an end-of-life suite—these are private rooms for mothers like me who were having stillborn babies or babies where there was low expectancy of the baby living outside the womb. The midwife, Sarah, who looked after me was lovely. She was my dedicated nurse on the ward while I was there to give birth. I felt very safe with her.

A doctor came in and gave me prostaglandin starting at 1 p.m., which would be administered every four hours. After the first pessary, I had some cramping and back pain. They checked and I had not dilated yet. My husband stayed with me and then went home for dinner after my sister and my mother arrived to be with me. He returned that evening and stayed the night with me.

They administered the second pessary near 6 p.m. Not much happened after, just more mild cramping, back pain and I was given IV paracetamol. The staff on the ward checked me again at 10:30 p.m. and I was 1 cm dilated. They then administered a third pessary. The cramping and back pain continued. I asked for more pain relief and got IV paracetamol, which did help with the pain, thankfully. My sister and I watched an online streaming service for most of the evening. She left and then my husband and I tried to sleep from 11:30 p.m.

At 3:45 a.m., I was still 1 cm dilated, but my cervix had thinned—which they explained was progress too. They gave me a fourth pessary which brought on some stronger contractions. I asked for more serious pain relief, and they gave me pethidine and IV paracetamol at 4:30 a.m. They checked my cervix again as the pain had increased, but apparently, my cervix was still at 1 cm but looking thinner. The medication gave me relief but only for an hour, allowing me to get a bit of sleep, thankfully.

At 6 a.m. I woke up to more intense pain and felt a sort of popping sensation. My waters had broken, which brought on more discomfort. I went into the loo, as I had a sensation like I just needed to sit. It felt like bad cramping you would have with diarrhea, but way more intense. We called the staff and at 6:20 a.m. they checked my cervix again. I was 3 cm dilated and my contractions were coming strong and fast at that point. There was maybe a minute between them. It was go time. The midwives put me into a wheelchair and brought me downstairs to the birthing suite between the contractions. The trip down was a bit of a blur as the contractions continued to get stronger.

I was given gas and air once in the labor suite and I got onto all fours every time I had a contraction. I found it very hard to use the gas and air. The midwives were encouraging me to use it and I kept refusing for some reason. I felt like I could not slow my breathing and was roaring my way through each contraction shouting, "No! No! No!"

We were waiting on the anesthesiologist to get to the ward and administer an epidural. He didn't show for what seemed like a very long time. I was just trying to deal with each contraction. The midwives wanted to examine me but the contractions were so close together that I couldn't sit still for them. The anesthesiologist arrived eventually and kept asking me to sign the consent form. I only had about ten or fifteen seconds between contractions at that point. As he put the form in front of me, I felt another contraction and the strong urge to push. After the next contraction, I managed to sign the form.

At that point, my husband and the team were telling me that I had to get into a seated position and had to stay perfectly still to allow the anesthesiologist to administer the epidural. The midwives were able to check again and I was 10 cm dilated. I could feel that Lily was crowning, but I was so determined to get the epidural that I did not care! The epidural was administered, although it did not have the full effect before it was time for me to push. The midwives got me onto my back with my feet in stirrups. I was roaring with each push and the midwife told me to press my lips together and push three big pushes. Lily was soon out, born at 7:30 a.m.

I think I was actively in labor for about forty minutes. It was so quick and I was in awe of my body and its amazing ability to do exactly what it needed to do. I was grateful for the mercy of a rapid labor under such devastating circumstances. I had been under the impression that there could be challenges with labor and delivery for those in a fat body. I am so proud of my body and what it was able to do.

After Lily was born, I delivered the placenta. I remember just getting through each step, from one to the next and then the aftermath—dealing with the death of my firstborn child. I remember the silence in the room— no cry and no squirming baby. The midwives asked if I wanted to hold her. I was so afraid. They encouraged me and I held her in my arms. She was quite damaged where her skin had become very fragile. This is a normal aspect of delivering a stillborn baby. I stared at her and held her little hand. She was my first and she was so beautiful and still.

My mum and sister arrived and my husband, mum and sister all took turns holding her. It was both sad and lovely. The midwives then dressed Lily and with clothes and a hat on, she just looked like she was sleeping in the cutest little onsie covered in monsters. Lily was 9 lbs 2 oz and 61 cm tall. She was such a big, healthy-looking baby.

We got to keep her in the room with us in a special cooled cot called a "cuddle cot" supplied by a charity called *Feileacain*. The charity also gave us a memory box with a baby blanket and other items, which were a huge comfort. The midwives who looked after us from the day we went in to hear the bad news, to the day we left with Lily were amazing, kind people with so much compassion. We will never forget them and will carry Lily with us forever in our hearts.

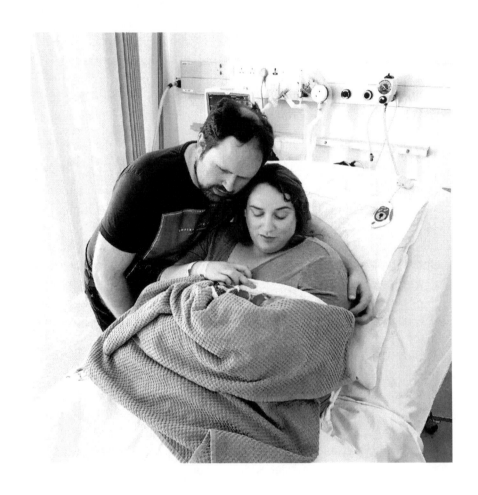

Julie Cook, Wales:

This was my third pregnancy, second baby, and I immediately knew I wanted a home birth. I didn't take much positivity away from the hospital birth of my son and I aimed for things to be different this time. Don't get me wrong—I had no complications during labor with him and delivered him on a hospital bed using gas and air, but the healing afterwards was horrendous. I had a second-degree tear and a labial tear that was not stitched. The pain I experienced as a result was the worst pain I had ever felt in my life. It was to the point of my mental health suffering and bonding with him was delayed.

This time there was no question about where I wanted to birth. All through my pregnancy I said that my dream birth would be at home with just me and my husband and have him deliver the baby. I did not think this would happen, though, and assumed the midwives would be there. I prepared my birth plan and said I wanted as little involvement from the midwives as possible, my husband to catch the baby and announce the sex. We chose not to find out the sex this time and it was fab. I had a stress-free pregnancy and no issues other than symphysis pubis dysfunction (SPD) towards the end.

The 22nd arrived and there was no sign of baby. I was disappointed, as I always assumed they would arrive early. Then I remembered that my original due date had been the 25th and just assumed that it would be closer to that date. I had a midwife appointment on the 25th just for a checkup and a chat. That morning I felt unwell with a migraine coming on and tired. My husband came home from work early and took me to my appointment. All went well and I returned home to nap for a few hours.

During the day, I had on-and-off pains in my back and lower stomach. I did not think much of them as I suffered with pains from the SPD anyway. As the day went on, they continued and eventually by 9 p.m., I thought they might genuinely be contractions. My husband and I went to bed as normal and were about to go to sleep when the pains started coming every ten minutes. We decided to go downstairs, get everything ready and start timing them. We watched a movie, had a cuppa and chilled out. I kept timing the contractions and they were all over the place.

They started coming every five minutes, then ten and thirty. During this time I used the TENS machine, which helped to distract me from the discomfort. I tried using my yoga ball but that didn't feel comfortable, so I just sat on the sofa instead. As it was approaching 3 a.m., I kept needing to urinate after each contraction and decided at that point that it would be a while until baby arrived. I went to the toilet again at 3:10 a.m., and that was when I noticed my mucus plug coming away.

The contractions started coming every two minutes as I shouted downstairs for my husband to phone the labor ward and to send the midwives to the house. At this point I could not move from upstairs—I just kept thinking I needed to pee all the time! My husband said the community midwife was going to call him back and I thought maybe she would arrive soon so I could have some gas and air towards the end. The contractions started to increase in their intensity, and they had already been pretty intense from the start. That was when I realized there was no time at all and the baby was going to arrive very soon.

My breathing changed and I began to moo. This was it—no pain relief. This baby was coming! I stood at the bottom of the bed breathing deep and mooing through the contractions. My waters started leaking and my husband quickly took off my underwear. I kept asking where the midwife was and saying the baby was coming, so my husband phoned the labor ward again. He kept them on speaker phone as I felt the baby coming down and bob back up. I started shouting that the baby was coming and there was no time.

The lady on the phone instructed me to get on all fours on the floor, as it would be easier than standing. I got down and the lady asked my husband what he could see. He said he was not sure—the room was quite dark as only one bedside lamp was on. He said he thought he saw the cord when the baby bobbed down again.

During this time I was focusing on getting the baby to crown—not that I had a choice! My body completely took over and was pushing by itself. Suddenly, I managed to get over the last hurdle and baby crowned. I reached between my legs to feel the head, which was surreal. My husband was still talking to the lady on the phone as she was instructing him what to do. The crowning was the part I feared most, but a calm came over me and I talked through what I was doing.

I breathed baby's head out and the remaining waters followed, which was such a relief. I knew with the next contraction my baby would be here. I remember saying out loud, "It's okay—with the next contraction, I'll push the body out." I could hear the baby making a little cry from between my legs and then with the next contraction, I pushed.

My husband had a towel ready to catch but the pressure made me think he was pushing the baby back in! I gave him a row and then realized it was just the force of the baby coming out! Baby arrived immediately after and my husband kept saying, "He's here! Oh my God, he's here!" and trying to rub him in mid-air.

The lady on the phone asked whether it was a boy or girl and because my husband had said "he," I thought we had another son. I peered through my legs as my husband was checking and saw that it was a girl! I was so happy, as I knew all along she was a girl. Eventually, I got up and brought my leg over the long umbilical cord and I held her skin to skin. She arrived at exactly 4 a.m.

The midwife arrived twenty minutes later as I sat on the bed in disbelief at what had just happened. It was the most amazing birth and my husband really was the best "midwife". He took me by surprise. I waited another fifty minutes for my placenta to come out naturally whilst my husband had a chat and a cuddle with our daughter on the landing.

Ivy Grace weighed 7 lbs 3 oz and was 51 cm long—the image of her daddy and brother. Her birth was my dream birth, everything that I wanted.

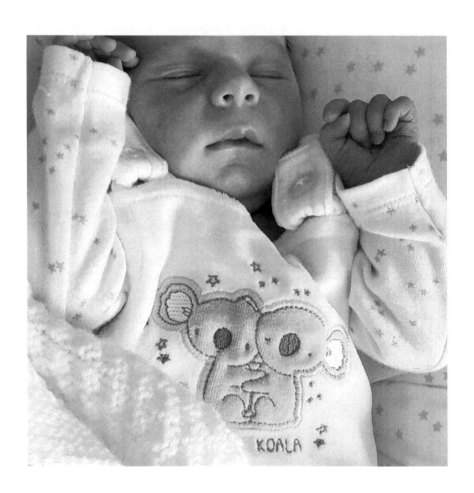

Rosie, UK:

I found out I was pregnant in February 2020 and my baby girl was born on October 27th. I was already having growth scans because of my BMI and it was then I was told my baby's estimated birth weight was 7 lbs 15 oz. This predicted weight plus my gestational diabetes diagnosis at thirty-seven weeks meant induction was discussed. We decided to go ahead and booked it for thirty-eight weeks and six days.

The induction process began with a pessary being inserted at 10:30 p.m. on Sunday. My husband was there for the pessary being inserted and then was asked to leave. I started getting Braxton Hicks contractions and they continued all night. At 8 a.m. the next morning, the midwives attached the monitors and told me baby was fine. The monitor had started picking up the tightening sensations I was feeling—about six within ten minutes. I was not feeling them as contractions, just my uterus hardening and lifting.

After I enjoyed a shower, the midwife was waiting to hook me up to do four hours of continuous fetal monitoring. Literally within two minutes of being hooked up, the machine started alarming because Wren's heartbeat had spiked. The pessary was then removed and my cervical dilation checked—I was 2 cm. The midwives then put a cannula in to rush some fluids through to baby. Whilst they were doing that, my baby's heart rate then dropped to the other end of the scale and was not being picked up by the machine at all! I was quickly transferred over to the labor ward at 11 a.m., which felt very frantic and frightened me. By the time they got us hooked back up to the drip and the monitor, her heartbeat was fine.

The contractions continued coming and I was really feeling them now, having to use "up breathing" to get through. My midwife needed the opinion of doctors who were all in theater and then there was a shift change. I managed until 3 p.m. by breathing through the contractions and then was offered to have my waters released. I accepted and then my dilation was assessed—3 cm. From 11 a.m. to 3 p.m. I had been continuously monitored and my belongings were left way out of my reach. I did not have access to my speaker, my nice electric tealight candles, my room spray or snacks. In hindsight, I should have rung the bell to have someone get them for me, but I was worried I would be told I was not "allowed". I decided to focus on sleep instead.

My husband was permitted in at this point. It was tough being without him, especially when things had been a bit scary that morning. He had already driven to and from the hospital a few times that morning and waited outside for a few hours just in case. I was so pleased to see him. He immediately got the room set up the way we wanted with the fake candles and familiar smells. Nothing changed with the contractions and no waters seemed to appear either. At 3:30 p.m., the midwife tried to see if releasing my waters had worked. It turns out Wren's head was blocking my cervix and thus, my waters from coming out. Once her head moved, my waters came out like a waterfall—just like what you see in movies!

We were given about fifty minutes after the waters released to let things progress naturally before we would need to think about going to the hormone drip. They needed some blood from me first in case I ended up having an epidural. It took two midwives and three attempts each for them to finally get some blood out of me. The contractions did not intensify at all so I accepted the drip and made the decision to have the epidural with it—best decision ever!

I went straight from the "up breathing" technique to epidural and never tried any pain relief between. The epidural meant I could stop focused breathing through the contractions and sleep a bit. Another reason I chose it was because we were not sure how Wren would react to the drip, based on her reaction to the pessary and the fact that I never stopped having four to six contractions every ten minutes.

The epidural and catheter were inserted at 6:30 p.m. when my cervix was 3 cm dilated. I was unfortunately given an epidural machine which kept intermittently stopping the top-ups being administered. This meant I experienced contractions having no idea how intense they would be. The epidural kept wearing off in one area so I did keep needing the top-ups. That was tough and I wobbled at one point because I couldn't prepare properly. Eventually, the midwife managed to get a password for the machine, so she could operate it without always having to rely on the anesthesiologist every time.

At midnight, Wren's heart rate did the same thing it had that morning— it shot through the roof and disappeared again. My midwife was using both her hands to keep the monitors in place on my belly when she told my husband to push the big, red emergency button. My room literally filled with people and a doctor placed an internal fetal monitor on my baby's head. I was told this was easier monitoring and that I was now 6 cm dilated.

I had another exam at 4 a.m. when I was 9 cm, with just a small cervical lip left. I reached full dilation at 5:30 a.m. Our midwife mentioned she probably wouldn't get to see our baby be born, as the shift change was at 7:15 a.m., which we were all a bit sad about.

Due to having an epidural, they gave me an hour to wait before pushing to give baby a chance to get used to the new contractions and move down. I lay on my side which was much better than being on my back. It was not as good as being up on all fours or another upright position, but I couldn't feel my legs! I could feel my baby moving down with every contraction during this hour and actually thought she was going to birth herself. I was sure if my husband looked he would see her face staring back because she felt that low.

The epidural had more than partially worn off and I was instructed to start pushing at 6:30 a.m. Within three contractions, I felt her face coming out, followed by her whole head and the rest of her body. My husband watched and said, "Her head is born! I'm looking at her!"

She was trying to cry already when she only had her head out! She was born and placed on my belly at 6:36 a.m. I did not have any tears or grazes anywhere, which I was happy about. It was beautiful with just me, my husband, our midwife (who managed to be present for the birth after all) and baby Wren with our electric tealight candles and playlist on in the background.

I reflect back on my birth in a hugely positive way. I felt empowered by having the vaginal birth and like a superhero for having no episiotomy or tears. I would do it all again tomorrow and only wish that it were possible. I cannot wait to share this story with my daughter.

Baby girl Wren was born on October 27th, 2020—7 lbs 14 oz. So much for my "giant" baby!

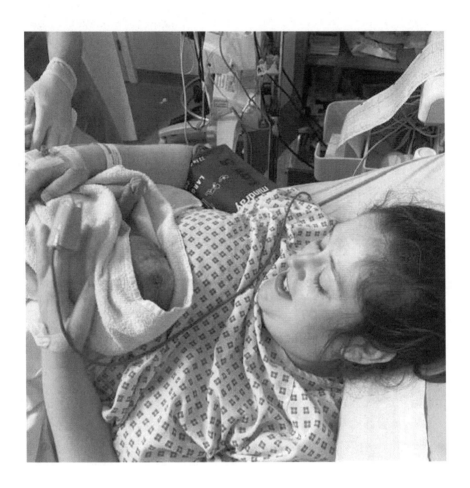

Christina Hughes, United States:

** Content warning for weight stigma in a medical setting.

I am a fat person. Always have been and always will be. The first time I ever told a care provider I wanted to be a mom, they told me (at age fourteen) that I would have to lose weight first.

It is a complicated story, but the short version is that I, myself, was premature at birth. This caused some developmental issues with my reproductive organs and my fallopian tubes were actually attached incorrectly. I required emergency surgery to fix this and allow me to begin my cycle. Because of this, I saw gynecologists a lot younger than many and had a lot more procedures, exams and surgeries... and a lot more fatphobia too.

Although I did not recognize it as such, I was shamed for my weight by care providers from that very first appointment. It continued until I found my midwife who helped me bring my daughter into this world. Why is this relevant to my birth story? Because of these experiences, my whole life I believed that being a mom was predicated on thinness, would take forever and would be made more difficult because of my size.

For fifteen years I tried to be skinnier, for a lot of reasons engrained by diet culture, but mostly because I wanted to be a mom. I was scared out of my mind that if I could not shrink myself, I would never achieve that desire.

In case you find any similarities in your story, I am here to tell you this: IT WAS BULLSHIT.

Weighing 255 lbs and ending my pregnancy around 300, I conceived within two months of "trying," carried and birthed a beautifully healthy baby girl with zero labor interventions. I birthed vaginally and unmedicated in a birthing pool in my bedroom—exactly how I wanted to.

The fear of being fat and pregnant influenced so many decisions around pregnancy and birth; it affected when I chose to start trying to conceive, how I considered, my worthiness of becoming a mom and led to disaster trains of thought about how my labor and delivery would go. About three years prior to becoming pregnant, I had started exploring diet culture, body positivity, listening to a few podcasts and changing the way I thought about the once dreaded "F word." I had come to accept my larger body enough and gave her some props, some of the time. I stumbled across the HAES (health at every size) movement and started reading things by Lindo Bacon. Slowly, over time, I started to hate my body a little less each day and I began thanking her for what she had gotten me through thus far. I would not say I loved my body then, nor do I fully love her now, but I did embrace her.

Fast forward to when my husband and I decided that we wanted to start trying to conceive. Even though I was more on the body acceptance train, I was still convinced that pregnancy would be long and awful and labor would be horrible and painful—mostly because I was fat. My fat body did get some credit because I got pregnant so quickly, something the doctors told me would take at least a year. But at this point, I had not experienced any change in my beliefs about my ability to actually birth a baby. I was still terrified of that event. I was fearful that my body would "fail me", and I would have another trauma to add to my list. I still held the deep belief that my big, fat body could not possibly see me through birth—that joyful, positive pregnancies and births were experiences reserved only for thin people.

Again… bullshit.

While I cannot tell you I had a clear "a-ha moment" where everything changed, there was a definite point early in my pregnancy when I heard a little voice say *it doesn't have to be this way.*

And, for the first time in a long time, I listened. I chose to believe that my story would be different. I started furiously trying to find other stories about fat pregnant people who had positive births. I started researching about body mass index and pregnancy as I enfolded fat-friendly language into my daily life. I interviewed potential care providers about their practices to try and sniff out any fat shaming. I decided that I would do everything I could to trust my body, listen to her, thank her and experience the whole damn thing just as I was supposed to. I decided that my pregnancy and birth would be for me and not anyone else.

And so, for the next eight months, I continued therapy, journaled, listened to meditations, researched, read, listened to podcasts, posted affirmations around the house and I hired a doula who was very familiar with fat bodies and served clients of all shapes. This self-work was the preparation that changed not only my labor and delivery but how I continue to show up for myself—and my daughter— every day.

One of the true testaments to the belief in my strength occurred around thirty-six weeks when baby was still breech. The OB who reviewed my ultrasound told me that meant I needed to schedule a cesarean. This was not a course I wanted to take. I took the information back to my midwife and asked what my options were. She confirmed it was a cesarean unless baby turned or we had a successful external cephalic version (ECV). An ECV, where a doctor manually turns the baby from the outside of your body, attempts to keep a baby head down and avoid a cesarean or vaginal breech birth. This was possibly one of the most intense and painful things I experienced my whole pregnancy, including labor. Luckily for us, it worked and was worth it.

Now, the nitty-gritty… I was lucky to be able to use vacation time and I took about a week off prior to my actual due date. I did not want to be commuting to work and I wanted to relax, especially after the copious nesting that took place. About three days before my due date, I started having mild contractions. They felt like small stomach cramps at first and over time progressed, growing in intensity and length. After about forty-eight hours with very little sleep, no water breaking, lots of calls to my midwife asking her if it was time, things started to get more intense. My doula arrived first and helped us set up the birth pool and labor in different positions.

Once the midwives arrived and set up, they asked to check how far along I was. Much to their surprise, I was almost 7 cm dilated. At this point, my cervix was not fully effaced and baby girl was not 100 percent in the right position. For this reason, I did some laboring with side lunges, involving my leg on a stool to try and get her and my cervix fully ready.

And my oh my, did that work! All I remember is this shift to insane pressure. I felt like I needed to poop and like my whole vagina was going to explode. That sounds graphic, but it is the best way I can describe it. It was not painful like when you hurt yourself, but just a whole lot of pressure where I had never felt pressure before. The contractions picked up to a quick pace with only about twenty to thirty seconds between them. It was difficult to find my breath and composure at times, but your mind really does go someplace else. They talk about "labor land" and I had definitely arrived.

I was back in the pool at this point and the primal noises came in full force. I found a rhythm that I focused on so intently that I literally cannot tell you what happened or how long that carried on. I used positive affirmations and counting my breath silently in my head, while my husband and doula were supporting me physically. Were there moments where I thought I could not keep going? Hell yes—I was so tired of the pressure, it was so strong and strange and I was just plain tired after three days of some form of laboring. (We later discussed that this pressure was probably because my waters never broke. My daughter was born en caul, still inside the intact amniotic sac—so the full pressure of her and the waters were on my pelvis).

At around 11:55 a.m. I looked at the clock and thought one more time, How am I going to keep going? I have no idea how much longer this is going to be! I remember blurting out some less sophisticated version of this thought in a breathy more panicked voice, "I can't do this if it gets any harder! Please tell me it's not going to be harder!" The whole team reassured me that my body was doing what it was supposed to and that it was not going to get harder, it was going to change. Somehow that was reassuring and I returned to labor land, albeit briefly.

At that moment, the sensation of the pressure changed 180 degrees and it vanished. It was replaced with this sensation of a deep feeling and she was definitely ready to come earth side. The timeline I kept running through my head was *thirty minutes to an hour, thirty minutes to an hour, and then I'll meet my baby.*

Not quite—I had seven minutes! I felt the pushing sensation three times: one of which I exclaimed, "I'm pushing," the second, "She's coming!" and the third, "She's here!" The midwives were scrambling around as I do not think anyone thought she would come so fast. They barely had time to put on their gloves and catch her in the pool. Her head came out and they told me not to push again, but there was no controlling that pushing—out she came!

The rest of the day was a magical blur. We got to do skin to skin, deliver the placenta, move into our cozy bed, feed and then do the newborn exam. We then took a huge nap as a family and woke up to start the adventure of raising our daughter, Remy Mei.

When I look back at this experience, the process was a transformation. I moved from a place of so much fear to a place of liberation from that fear and being in awe of my fat body that made, grew and brought my daughter into this world.

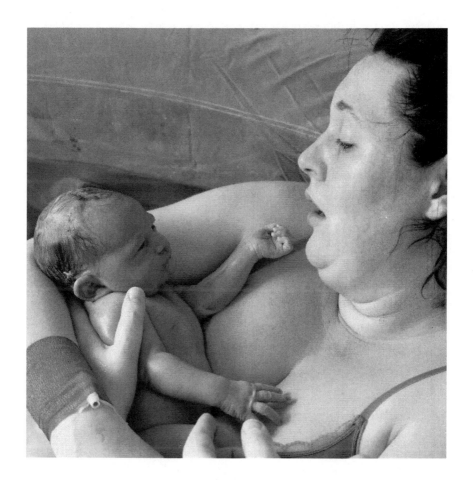

Stacey, Ireland:

*** Content warning for weight stigma in a medical setting.*

I found out I was pregnant just before Christmas of 2019. At only a few weeks along, I thought to myself *this is going to be a long pregnancy.* My happiness and joy quickly turned to fear and anxiety. I nervously did an online search for "fat and pregnant" and to my dismay, there weren't many positive stories. The results were all about how a higher BMI could lead to complications in pregnancy.

I booked an early pregnancy scan at eight weeks and took over six pregnancy tests, as I just couldn't believe it. On the drive to the scan center, all that was going through my head was *what if they cannot find the baby through my fat? What if my baby can't survive in there?* My partner and I were only waiting three minutes before we were called in. Within seconds of the ultrasound wand hitting my skin, there he was—my perfect little baby.

Filled with joy and positivity, for that day at least, my pregnancy went on with very little symptoms. Fatigue was my main complaint. In three week's time, I wasn't feeling well in general, but over the years I recognized the feeling as being overly stressed. I was in a stressful job that I had only begun the September before, so I was still finding my own feet.

When I had a check up with the doctor, my blood pressure was raised. This was not due to the baby at all but could affect the baby. The doctor gave me a few weeks off to try and settle the high blood pressure, although the consistent worrier in me made it impossible to relax. I was then put on high blood pressure tablets.

At my first booking scan at thirteen weeks, again, I was concerned about how they would see the baby and if he was okay. This time he was much bigger with a clearly visible head, body, legs and arms. He was just perfect. Due to my blood pressure being high on this occasion also, the doctor upped my medication and asked me to return to the clinic every month due to my pregnancy now being classed as "high-risk."

At the thirty week mark, my pregancy was going well and I had begun seeing a little difference in my belly. My baby was up high and he was kicking strongly. He would move around at night when I would lay down, and I could see my belly move. At each scan he was growing and the consultant kept telling me he was a big baby, measuring weeks ahead of his due date.

I was scanned every two weeks at the end of my pregnancy. I was always told that my baby would be big but that it would be, "No problem to ya because you're a big lady, too."

Although I took no offence to it, I found it funny how comfortable everyone was saying that to me. Due to the high blood pressure classing my pregnancy as high-risk, I was told I should have been induced two weeks before my due date. I met with one midwife who wasn't happy with the lack of a plan at the time. She sorted everything out and handed me a piece of paper with the induction date on it. I finally knew when I would meet my little man, but he had other plans.

I felt a sudden urge to run for the toilet at 1 pm. My waters had released, but there were no contractions. I was admitted onto the maternity ward at 2:30 pm with no change. The midwives did check on my baby and he was still happy inside. I was brought to a bed and told the doctors would make a plan of action in the morning.

At 9 am the following day, I was lucky to meet with an obstetrician who said, "Why wait? Let's induce you and get things rolling."

I was hooked up to a drip of Pitocin to induce my labor at 1 pm. Six hours later, the contractions I was experiencing were no worse than mild period pains. It was decided a cesarean was needed.

A bit of embarrassment washed over me as the hospital staff prepared me for the cesarean. I wondered if the surgery would be more challenging because of my size. I quickly pushed that aside when I thought about meeting my son. I got the epidural, lay flat on my back and the team got to work.

My son was lifted out at 9:02 pm and he began crying—and that was me done. I was crying, emotional, in love and anxious to hold him. As they continued to finish the surgery, my partner got to hold our son. There he was—the boy who immediately stole my heart. He didn't care what size his mammy was and I didn't care what size I was either.

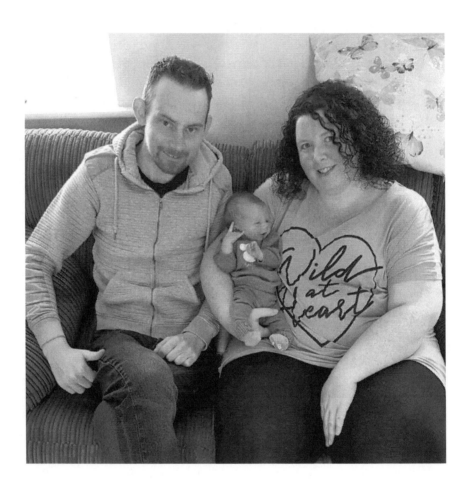

Dorita, England:

In 2014, I had an emergency cesarean during my first daughter's birth. When I became pregnant with my second daughter in 2019, I was adamant that I would do everything in my power to ensure that I had a successful vaginal birth after cesarean, a VBAC.

Unfortunately, every midwife appointment I attended was focused on my weight. This happened even though I was considerably lighter than I was during my first pregnancy. I was told that I would more than likely need to have an elective cesarean due to my weight and prior cesarean. My hope of having a VBAC seemed impossible when I was presented with that information.

Even though my blood pressure was fine at every appointment, the conversation was always about how my risks for preeclampsia and uterine rupture were increased due to my BMI. I was constantly being talked out of my wish for a VBAC. I began to dread seeing my midwives.

Eventually, I was seen by a doctor who gave me hope. He told me that my chances of a successful VBAC were approximately 60 percent and that if I wanted to go for it he was happy to support me. If it had been appropriate, I would have kissed the poor man there and then!

Seven days past my due date, I spontaneously went into labor and made my way to the hospital. I was told I was already 5 cm dilated and ready to go to the labor ward. Due to my previous cesarean, I had a cannula placed in my arm to make it easier for me to be taken to theater in case of a uterine rupture.

Thankfully everything progressed smoothly and my body seemed to take over and do what it needed to. After a few hours of labor, I finally felt the need to push and was encouraged to do so by the midwife.

I am not entirely sure how many pushes it took to get my daughter's head out, but it only took one involuntary push for the rest of her body to emerge.

My second daughter was born on November 21st, 2019—the morning of her big sister's fifth birthday. I had never been so happy and proud of myself and my body before. My body is capable of great things.

Gabrielle Gill, United States:

** Content warning for weight stigma in a medical setting.

"You should probably take a pregnancy test. You're being way more bitchy than usual," I said to Samantha, my sister, as we made plans to meet up for breakfast that December morning.

"I'm not pregnant but bring one just in case," she said, telling me to hurry up because she was already on her way.

I glanced over at my own pregnancy test sitting on the bathroom window ledge. I was not late yet, as I expected my period to start that day. I had spotted the night before but curiously woke up to a dry liner. I had successfully practiced the fertility awareness method for two years, but the reassurance of bulk-ordered pregnancy tests was always welcomed.

Oh good, negative—I thought to myself as I spotted it across the bathroom. I went to toss it, and there it was—ever so faint. Was it even there? Did I remember to put my contacts in? I squinted. Barely there, it looked like a shadow of the line next to it—*Eh, must be a fluke.*

I'll just take another since that one is defective, I thought smartly. It truly did not occur to me that it could be positive. I sent a picture to Samantha who immediately called me. "BITCH YOU'RE PREGNANT!"

The brain is incredible. I graduated from an Ivy League midwifery program, I see hundreds of patients a week and if this were one of their tests in the office, I would have told them they were pregnant. Yet looking at my two tests, I remained in disbelief—even after I took four or five more. I made my sister stop and get me a digital test on her way and that one really was defective, as it stayed blank! It was not until its replacement blinked "Pregnant" that I began to process the word in a whole new way. Then my knees hit the porcelain bathroom tile, which would soon become their new resting place. I promptly dry-heaved and broke out into a full-body sweat. "What? How? Where—?"

China. My husband and I had been on vacation for ten days the previous month. We had left the morning after a twenty-four-hour shift at the hospital and with the lack of sleep, jet lag and time change, I made an error in my tracking. Just the night before at dinner with Samantha, she had asked Andrew and when we were having kids.

"Not any time soon, if ever," I said confidently as I sipped my white

Russian.

Well, I guess "ever" was here. *And shit, did I already mess this baby up? No, I'm only three weeks and three days along, no damage done. Ok, but how embarrassing for a midwife to get accidentally pregnant.* I had only been married and at this new job for six months. This wasn't "The Plan."

Now that he is here and I am so deeply in love with my son, I cannot believe I ever felt this way. I was not sad—part of me was excited but I felt so many other things.

I did not get to have the naiveté many new mothers have with their first pregnancy due to my profession. I was afraid to get attached to my baby—afraid I would lose him and would not recover. I had seen so many parents' worst days. I went to my familiar comfort zone of distancing my feelings and focusing on logistics. I did not really bond with my baby until my third trimester. My midwife brain was gone—I knew that pregnancy was normal and healthy the majority of the time. I also knew that a "baby blues" time during the first trimester was common, even among people who have tried for years to conceive—but that did not stop my guilty. I felt for not being "capital H happy" and for getting pregnant easily and accidentally when my coworkers and friends struggled and suffered losses.

When I was able to lift my head from the toilet following twenty-seven weeks of nausea, I became intentional about making as safe a space as I could for my plus size pregnancy and myself. Yes, I am a large-bodied gal, but I had no health problems and my risks of a few things were only slightly increased. I followed every fat or body positive pregnancy account I could. Flooding my feed with pictures of women who looked like me, with bellies that looked like mine, helped normalize my experience. It was also a salve to the fatphobic comments I constantly heard at work—comments about other women in large bodies that were said to me in an attempt to make conversation. "Well, I mean she is 300 pounds and it's all in her stomach; that kid isn't coming out."

I would rehearse how I would react the next time I heard one of these comments, but every time I froze. My blood boiled and my eyes would get hot—why say these things at all but especially to me?

Aside from vomiting myself to unintentional weight loss, which I was, of course, commended for, I had a medically uncomplicated pregnancy. Eventually, I did respond to fatphobic comments directed towards me and, horrifyingly, even my unborn baby!

Time seemed to fly when I was pregnant. I went to the chiropractor, pelvic floor physical therapist and took daily walks.

My second trimester gave me the famous burst of energy. I remodeled my dining room and stripped and painted our dining table. I planned out and made a backyard garden that only got half planted due to symphysis pubis pain. I took hypnobirthing classes online and forced myself to meditate and read parenting books.

One of my favorite memories was the late nights spent listening to Harry Potter audiobooks or podcasts as I painted the epic-themed nursery mural my talented husband had drawn on the walls. I was starting to get so excited to show this kid a magical world, both the one that lives in pages and the one we can discover ourselves. I started planning to take a trip in August every year to celebrate our birthdays. All of a sudden, I found myself really looking forward to meeting this kid, but not too soon—I had a lot to do!

I had always wanted a home birth, but there were no Certified Nurse Midwives (CNM) providing home births in my area. There were Certified Practicing Midwives in the state of Maryland, but their licenses do not allow them to attend home births for women with a BMI over thirty-five. This was beyond upsetting, as a pregnant woman and a CNM. Had I just bought my house ten minutes north in Delaware or ten minutes south in Virginia, I would have been able to have a home birth as the scope of practice of midwives in those states takes in the overall health of the woman and does not place a cap on BMI. Luckily, I love my midwife coworkers and there are many phenomenal nurses and skilled doctors at my job, so I planned a low intervention hospital birth there.

When I was thirty-eight weeks, I had unprecedented stress levels at work and I began having irritable bowel syndrome symptoms that I had not experienced in nearly a decade. The intestinal cramps triggered uterine contractions and I lost ten pounds in a week. I worked my last busy shift when I was thirty-eight weeks and the next day I had an intense urge to nest. My irritable intestines and uterus slowed me down, so Andrew and I stayed up most of the night as I decided the entire house needed to be rearranged. This was the night before we had to be up for our 4 a.m. sunrise maternity photo shoot. The next morning at 5 a.m., I waddled on the sand breathing through contractions trying to look relaxed and goddess-like. My stomach had dropped from its cute high position to the about-to-pop look that makes everyone around you a little nervous. I survived the photo shoot and went back home to finish my quest to flip my house.

I was standing in the doorway of the nursery, having just put something away, when I felt fluid run down my legs. I jolted—*it couldn't be, maybe this is just a lot of urine sneaking out.* Then came a waterfall of meconium fluid, which is a little unusual at thirty-eight weeks. Sometimes it can be a sign of fetal distress. I tried to stay calm and told my husband, who started running around packing random things in a bag. My midwife-friend, Rose, came over while he was getting things together and confirmed what I already knew. My membranes had ruptured, I was barely contracting and I was only 1 cm dilated.

When we arrived at the hospital, my co-workers had lovingly set up a room on the quiet end of the unit, had the lights dim and twinkly lights strung up. I was planning an unmedicated birth so we started using the breast pump to try to bring on a better contraction pattern. It worked, but they would stop as soon as it came off. My nipples got sore and I was exhausted, at 2 cm.

With teary eyes, I told Rose to start the Pitocin. I knew my risk of infection was going up and it would be harder to labor without pain relief. I could not bear the thought of being separated from my baby if we did get an infection.

The Pitocin began and my body responded quickly and hard. Suddenly, the contractions were on top of each other and I was not getting a break. I labored in every position I had ever seen or studied, but nothing helped. They were right on top of each other. The Pitocin got turned off, then back on, and I could not get on top of them. I had no energy left, I was delirious from lack of sleep and I had not eaten a meal in over a week because of my IBS. I tried the IV meds, which made me feel woozy and care less about the contractions for what felt like twenty minutes. I tried playing, my hypnobirth meditation track that I had listened to every day for most of my pregnancy, and for the first time, it irritated me. I couldn't stand it when I was having a contraction. I did use some techniques that helped me stay calm and present during this whole process, but it had been almost twenty-four hours and I knew I was far from delivery. What I was doing wasn't working—I needed to do something else. As the sun was going down, I opted for an epidural.

I did not like the way the epidural made me feel. My whole lower half was pins and needles and if I touched my own leg, it felt like I was touching someone else's. It freaked me out. I remember asking why patients don't talk about that more. It had only been in for one or two hours when I had this intense pressure in my butt and once again, I do not know where my midwife brain went. It never occurred to me to have someone check my cervix. I just assumed my epidural was not covering that area. I had just gotten checked right after my epidural was placed and it was 3 cm. I thought there was no way I had made a lot of change.

Rose came in to check my cervix before leaving for the night. She checked my cervix and then she started crying, asking me if I was ready to have a baby! Within a few hours I was fully dilated and baby was at zero station, which is why I felt so much pressure. My husband had left the hospital to get his medications he had forgotten, so I called him. It felt like it took forever for him to get back. I was so excited and everything felt lighter, hopeful and I was ready to meet my baby.

When he returned, everyone was getting ready, and without me knowing he snapped a picture of me. He posted it on social media announcing we were about to have a baby. I did not, see it until afterward but there were so many comments like, "She is going to kill you," "Did she say you could post this?"

I did not, but it seemed they were all saying those things because they thought it was a bad picture. My body was somewhat exposed and I looked like a fat woman about to give birth. I later wrote a long paragraph in response to their comments. I was glad he posted that picture. He was excited and it shows a plus size man watching his plus size wife about to have a very normal and healthy birth after a normal, healthy pregnancy. I wish I had seen more pictures of women of size giving birth when I was pregnant.

I had an amazing birth team and I felt comfortable and supported. I asked for my epidural to be turned off, as I was worried I would not feel to push—and I did not but somehow pushed in the right spot. My baby boy was here quickly and there is a picture of me looking into a mirror as he was crowning, smiling. Afterward, I thought, *well, you didn't make it unmedicated but you got your vaginal delivery and hey, it's kinda nice you didn't feel the ring of fire.*

I reached down and brought my baby to my chest. He was covered in vernix, had squishy cheeks and felt so familiar. I had the same feeling meeting him as I had on my first date with his dad. I thought, *oh here you are. I've always known you and you belong with me forever.*

My husband says he immediately saw me change and my instincts kick in. I know what he means—I was still myself, but I knew now things would always be different. I had prepared my husband and myself that there was a chance I would not bond right away with the baby, but that could not have been further from the truth. I was in love. I stayed up all night staring at him, in awe and wonder. Amazed that here he was, he was mine and we had made him.

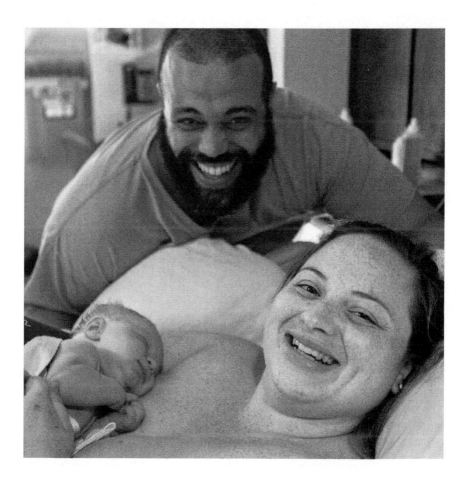

Annika, Germany:

During my entire pregnancy, I was really lucky and pleased with my medical support team. My gynecologist never commented on my weight or BMI, which I appreciated.

When I was twenty weeks pregnant, I was diagnosed with both high blood pressure and gestational diabetes. It was part of a routine checkup and I was glad it was discovered. I was referred to a specialist and instructed to measure my blood pressure three times a day. In the beginning it was really hard to change my diet mid-pregnancy, especially as an eating disorder survivor. Thankfully, I managed to get my blood sugar levels under control with the help and support of my husband—who is also an amazing cook.

It was important for me to recognize that there is no shame in developing gestational diabetes or high blood pressure. Contrary to what many people believe, developing these conditions may be down to hormones and not your body type. I was very happy with all of my medical team's treatment throughout my pregnancy. Two people did make comments about my weight, however, both of them were men that did not have anything to do with my pregnancy per se. They recommended that I should breastfeed my baby, "Because you will lose weight quicker then"— as if that was the main reason someone would want to breastfeed! Aside from those two people, my team was professional, competent and kind. I always felt safe with them.

I decided to get an induction based on my two risk factors. My baby and I were so healthy that the induction was scheduled for just two days before her estimated birth date. I arrived at the hospital on Christmas Day feeling a bit frustrated. I had hoped so much that I would not need to get an induction, as I heard so many horrible things—especially for plus size women.

My induction started and for the first thirty hours, nothing happened. I was not in pain, but being in a hospital over Christmas, missing my husband and playing the "waiting game" very frustrating for me.

At 11 p.m., I received my seventh dose of medication, then had my normal CTG (fetal heart rate monitor) and went to bed. Twenty minutes later, at 12:50 a.m., I felt something like a massive kick but also a rip. *Could this be my waters releasing?* I got up and went to the toilet—sure enough, my pajamas were drenched!

In the labor and delivery department, they told me to get a CTG if my waters broke, so I did. Everything was fine, so they sent me back downstairs and told me to return at 7 a.m. to get my next dose of induction medicine. I already had a few contractions, but they did not get picked up by the machine.

I went back to my room and within a matter of minutes, the contractions became regular. First, every five minutes, then every three minutes— lasting about a minute in length. When the contractions happened every three minutes, I walked back up to the labor and delivery ward. They did another CTG but still could not see the contractions. They checked my cervix, which was completely effaced but only 1 cm dilated. I was sent downstairs again to maybe catch some sleep, but of course I could not sleep with contractions every several minutes!

Lying on the bed felt very unnatural, so I sat on the toilet and practiced the good, old "forward, upright and open" position. Oddly enough, sitting on the toilet of all places worked very well in strengthening the contractions while at the same time keeping them bearable. To stay in control of the pain, I inhaled and counted to know when the individual contractions would stop. I kept doing that and also walked up and down the hallways for the next three hours. It was almost 6 a.m. when I decided that I would not be able to stand this pain for ten more hours or more. I am a firm believer in choice, science and medicine, so I decided to ask for an epidural. I knew I could cope with the intensity for another hour or two, but I did not know how much longer labor would be. I wanted to be sure to save my strength. I walked to the labor and delivery unit again for what felt like the tenth time that night. I told the midwife that I did not know how to go on. She connected me to the CTG again, comforted me and left the room to get something.

The moment the door was closed, the worst contraction so far hit and I was surprised by its intensity. All the pressure in my lower belly pushed down and I could not keep quiet anymore. Another midwife came in, heard my surprised scream and said, "Okay, I'll check your dilation now and won't wait for the CTG."

She looked me and said, "Did you call your husband yet? Your baby will be here within the hour."

I was totally baffled. The other midwife grinned and said, "Correction— it's too late for an epidural now!" I had to grin at that, too. It was 6:18 a.m. when I called my husband, who rushed to the hospital.

My bed was wheeled into another room and the midwives asked me if I could walk three steps to whatever birthing method I wanted—the chair, the bed and another thing I cannot remember. At this point, I felt completely relaxed, but also did not know what to do. The kind midwife suggested lying on my side in the bed with one leg up. It's funny, because this position was the one I saw during a birth preparation class and thought, *I probably won't want to do that.* It looked uncomfortable. At the moment, however, it was the most natural and comfortable position for me.

My midwife was really nice and I immediately trusted her. She told me when to push and when not to, while also offering her shoulder to support my upper leg. After a few pushes, I turned around to the other side. My husband arrived at the hospital at 6:55 a.m., following a long drive. At that point, baby's head was already crowning! I am forever grateful that my husband could be present at the time of our baby's birth, although it was only for five minutes. Within two more pushes, our baby girl was born at 7 a.m. exactly.

My birth experience as a fat person was incredibly positive. I felt in control at all times. My obstetrician during pregnancy and the hospital's midwife during birth were absolutely wonderful. My birth was amazing—although also exhausting, but I can honestly say I would not mind giving birth again in the same hospital in western Germany.

Sarah, UK:

*** *Content warning for weight stigma in a medical setting.*

I am on the higher end of the BMI scale and as such, I am generally considered unable to have a straightforward pregnancy, labor and birth—at least according to all the health professionals I have come across during my pregnancies.

After my home birth plans for my first daughter ended up being a consultant-led induction, I was more determined than ever that my second labor would be very different. Most of my pregnancy went fairly smoothly. I had some morning sickness and I went to all the appointments deemed necessary for fat pregnant people: the healthy eating clinic and the gestational diabetes tests. Happily, there were no problems during my pregnancy other than the odd fairly obnoxious sonographer who complained that my weight was making their job more difficult while huffing and puffing through my scans.

I was already prepared for the battle facing me before I even attended any hospital appointments. My first daughter was 6 lbs 9 oz, a little small but nothing to worry about—but then she was forced into this world before she was ready. Her dad has a small build and perhaps, with some irony, I was only 2 lbs when I was born, so it did not worry me having a small baby.

My consultant hospital appointments began at thirty-two weeks and induction pressure started immediately. It was assumed that because I was plus size, I should be having a big baby—so the fact that my baby was not predicted to be 10 lbs seemed to be an indication to them that something must be wrong. At this point, I found the most amazing doula, called Sam, and she helped me understand that it was okay to ask questions and okay for me to say no. This time around, more than anything, I did not want the constant internal vaginal examinations that left me with an infection and to be honest, feeling slightly violated following my first birth.

I kindly but firmly informed them at each appointment that I would not be agreeing to induction, "just in case". At my thirty-five-week appointment with the senior midwife, I explained how I wanted a home birth with a back up plan of a midwifery-led unit. After a very lengthy discussion and an agreement to have an injection to help deliver the placenta, as apparently "all fat pregnant women bleed more," she agreed to help me with my home birth plans. I did not really mind about the injection, so was happy to agree.

At thirty-seven weeks, I was told baby was not growing at the same rate as before and very quickly my home birth plans disappeared. I did, however, get the consultant to write in my notes that I could access the midwifery unit to use the birthing pool, providing I could get myself in and out unaided.

At thirty-nine weeks, I was informed that the fluid around my baby had halved and that I needed to be induced immediately. I asked what the chances were that a mistake had been made and I was told that it was pretty high and that probably all was ok. I was also told I could not have the birth I wanted and I was made to feel like a naughty school girl; being told I could not leave the hospital until a senior consultant agreed it was ok for me to leave.

The senior consultant agreed that the previous junior consultant had been a bit heavy-handed with the comments and a bit premature with the diagnosis, however, they wanted me to come in daily for monitoring. I agreed to do this for a week, but at my next appointment, I stated that all these appointments were doing me more harm than good—I would see them in one week's time.

At forty weeks, I again refused induction. I was told surely it was more important to take home a "live baby" than have the birth I wanted. I was livid.

At forty-one weeks, baby had started to move slightly less and I was definitely ready for baby to be here after all the negative comments that had been put in my head. The anxiety meant I was having trouble sleeping. I called the hospital and agreed to an induction but that it was all to be on my terms. I wrote a birth plan with the help of my doula, hopefully covering all possibilities. I knew birth is unpredictable but this time I was determined to have at least some of my wishes fulfilled. I wanted to keep hold of some control over my own body.

On October 3rd, 2019 I went into the induction suite to begin. My doula and I made sure the midwives all read the birthing plan before anything began, as it included things like minimum internal exams and minimal monitoring.

The induction gel worked pretty well and the midwives all stuck to my agreement with no pushing. I do think that was partly due to Sam's presence and she definitely gave me the courage to stick with what I was comfortable with. When I was told that they would be breaking my waters, I stated that they could do this as soon as the birthing pool became available.

I would wait on the induction suite until then. At 3 a.m. on October 5th, a midwife came to the suite to get me and take me to the birth pool room to break my waters.

A consultant came in to introduce himself and said he understood I wanted a hands-off, as much as possible, labor and just wanted to say hello. He stated he would leave me alone unless necessary to intervene. My waters were released with ease and pretty quickly the contractions ramped up a notch. After a few dances to some good old Disney tunes and a few laps of the hallway, I informed the midwife she had better get the pool filled as this baby was coming soon.

The pool was a dream. Contractions were getting more intense but amazingly, totally manageable. If anything, they felt empowering like I was in total control. The midwife was very respectful and it was not long before my body began to push my little one out. With a roar, I birthed my baby into this world, completely unaided and without the need for any intervention. I felt incredible and to be honest, could not believe it. Unlike the drug-induced haze of my first labor, I can remember all the wonderful details of this birth. I felt like I could do anything. It was the most amazing, intense and empowering experience of my life. I had never believed a pain-free birth was possible until now. Intense? Yes—but not painful.

I picked my daughter up from the bottom of the pool, straight into my arms. We sat there in the warm water in just a bubble of love and support. I never did end up having that injection as my placenta decided to make an appearance just as I was getting out of the pool.

It was sad that it was necessary for me to have to say no so many times up until this point and to feel like I needed to justify all my decisions. I was lucky in that I was able to hire an amazing doula who gave me the confidence to trust myself and question when I did not want to agree to something.

My midwife was also incredible and allowed me to just be, and for the first time, I did not feel like the "fat pregnant woman." I was just a woman in labor, eager to meet her little one for the first time. It makes me sad that we are led to believe that we cannot birth unaided and that we are putting our babies at risk if we want to question the decisions of health professionals. They may be very good at what they do, but it is still my body and now I know the amazing things it can do if it is just left alone.

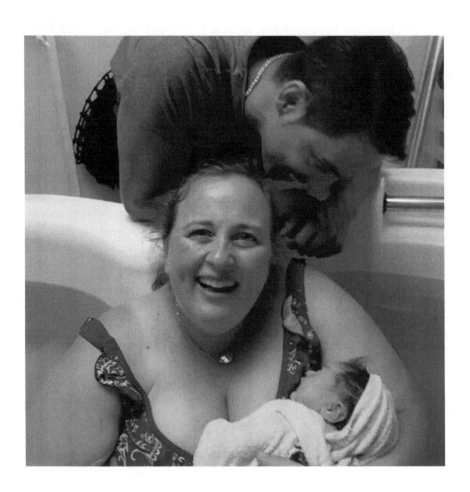

CONCLUSION: *You've Got This!*

Thank you so much for envisioning that fat pregnancy and birth can be experienced as something positive and beautiful—because they really can. Thank you for challenging the fatphobic status quo that is so heavily represented today. Each person who challenges these beliefs helps pave a more compassionate path for those who will give birth after us. Thank you for buying my book and believing in a dream that I have had since childhood. I put everything I have into these pages and I hope you have found them both accessible and helpful. You are wonderful. You are worthy. You are enough.

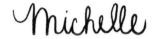

Further Resources

More from Michelle and Fat and Pregnant

Fat and Pregnant: www.fatandpregnant.com

Instagram: @fat.and.pregnant

Fat and Fertile by Nicola Salmon
Fearing the Black Body by Sabrina Strings
The F*ck It Diet by Caroline Dooner
Informed is Best by Amy Brown
More Than a Body by Lindsay and Lexie Kite
Trust Your Body, Trust Your Baby by Rosie Newman

WEBSITES

AIMS Ireland: www.aimsireland.ie
AIMS UK: www.aims.org.uk
Birth Monopoly: www.birthmonopoly.com
Birthrights UK: www.birthrights.org.uk
Dr. Sara Wickham: www.sarawickham.com
Dr. Sarah Buckley: www.sarahbuckley.com
Evidence Based Birth: www.evidencebasedbirth.com
Fat and Pregnant: www.fatandpregnant.com
Fat Positive Fertility Coach Nicola Salmon: www.nicolasalmon.co.uk
Improving Birth: www.improvingbirth.org
International Cesarean Awareness Network: www.ican-online.org
Kellymom Breastfeeding and Parenting: www.kellymom.com
La Leche League International: www.llli.org
NICE Guidelines: www.nice.org.uk
The VBAC Link: www.thevbaclink.com

BIBLIOGRAPHY

Crabbe, Megan Jayne. Body Positive Power: How to Stop Dieting, Make Peace with Your Body and Live. New York: Seal Press, 2018.

Dekker, Rebecca. Babies Are Not Pizzas: They're Born, Not Delivered! Evidence Based Birth, 2019.

Hill, Milli. Give Birth Like a Feminist: Your Body. Your Baby. Your Choices. London: HQ, 2019.

Orbach, Susie. Bodies. London: Profile Books LTD, 2010.

Resch, Elyse and Tribole, Evelyn. Intuitive Eating: a Revolutionary Program that Works. New York: St. Martin's Press, 2012.

Thomas, Laura. Just Eat It: How Intuitive Eating Can Help You Get Your Shit Together Around Food. London: Blue Books, 2019.

Acknowledgments

I have dreamt about becoming an author since I won my first writing award at the age of five. That first poem about a busy honey bee sparked the tiniest bit of confidence which I have been fueling and helping grow for almost three decades. There are so many people I have to thank who have supported me as I have journeyed from that unsure little girl to the woman (and author) I am now.

Thank you to my parents, siblings, extended family and friends who have supported me through the many ups and downs of life. A special thank you Mom and Dad for encouraging me to follow my dreams and write.

Thank you to my clients and thousands of supporters, both online and in-person. It is an honor to be invited along on your journey to becoming new parents.

I am so grateful for other birth advocates and fat activists who are shaking things up, fighting against oppressive policies and patriarchal systems. Thank you for creating waves and making change within the birth community and for fat people everywhere.

A large number of people have made this book practically possible and I am forever grateful. Thank you to my editors, Amber Hatch and everyone at Salt & Sage Books. Thank you to Charlotte Thomson-Morley for the cover design. Ashley Santoro has done the beautiful design and formatting for Fat Birth and I am so grateful! A massive thank you to all of the parents who contributed their birth stories and pictures for publication! Sharing a piece of your heart with the world is a big thing and I cannot thank you enough.

This book was also made possible through crowdfunding efforts via Kickstarter. Thank you to each and every person who contributed to my campaign, making the self-publication of *Fat Birth* possible. A special thank you goes out to Christina Hughes for supporting my project. Crowdfunding is a huge endeavor and it was only made possible with the help of videographer Tadhg Hayes and those who helped with the project rewards, including: Ashton Gelzinis, Caoimhe Walsh and Charlotte Thomson-Morley.

Thank you to the amazing community of women who provided me with loving, compassionate and respectful care as I birthed my own children: Jade Rayne, Madelaine Göhrs, Sandra Healy, Ann Bargh, Marta Korpys,

Natasha Vorozcova, Annika Schulz and Shelly O'Halloran. You all helped me understand how beautiful, vulnerable and powerful birth can be.

Lastly, my biggest thank you goes to my family for their loving support. My husband, Anthony—thank you for making me laugh every day and supporting my dreams. You have listened to me talk about this book for well over a year and I am grateful that you have been "my person" through it all. You have kept me going when overwhelm and self-doubt hit their hardest. To my wonderful children, Aidan, Niamh, William, Graham and Iris—thank you for understanding and allowing my passions to be part of our family life. I love you so much and I am so grateful you chose me to be your mommy.

Endnotes

INTRODUCTION

1. Evelyn Tribole and Elyse Resch, Intuitive Eating: a Revolutionary Program that Works. New York: St. Martin's Press, 2012, 76.

CHAPTER ONE

1. Chimamanda Ngozi Adichie, "The Danger of a Single Story," July 2009. TEDGlobal video, 18:33. https://www.ted.com/talks/chimaman-da_ngozi_adichie_the_danger_of_a_single_story

2. Sarah Slater, "Pregnant Women Allowing Themselves to Be Overweight is Criminal." Irish Examiner. July 25, 2018. https://www.irishexaminer.com/news/arid-30857587.html

3. Sean M. Phelan, J.I. Dovidio, R.M. Puhl, D.J. Burgess, D.B. Nelson, M.W. Yeazel, R. Hardeman, S. Perry, and M. van Ryn. "Implicit and Explicit Weight Bias in a National Sample of 4,732 Medical Students: the Medical Student CHANGES Study." Obesity (Silver Spring) 22, no. 4 (2014): 1201-1208. https://pubmed.ncbi.nlm.nih.gov/24375989/

4. Judy Anne Swift, S. Hanlon, L. El-Redy, R.M. Puhl, and C. Glazebrook. "Weight Bias Among UK Trainee Dietitians, Doctors, Nurses and Nutritionists." Journal of Human Nutrition and Dietetics 26, no. 4 (2013): 395-402. https://pubmed.ncbi.nlm.nih.gov/23171227/

5. Gregory Dodell. Quote from Instagram account Everything_Endocrine. Published February 16, 2021. www.instagram.com/everything_endocrine

6. A. Janet Tomiyama, D. Carr, E.M. Granberg, B. Major, E. Robinson, A.R. Sutin, and A. Brewis. "How and Why Weight Stigma Drives the Obesity 'Epidemic' and Harms Health." BMC Med 16, no. 123 (2018). https://doi.org/10.1186/s12916-018-1116-5

7. Sean M. Phelan, D.J. Burgess, M.W. Yeazel, W.L. Hellerstedt, J.M. Griffin, and M. van Ryn. "Impact of Weight Bias and Stigma on Quality of Care and Outcomes for Patients with Obesity." Obesity Reviews 16, no. 4 (2015): 319-326. https://pubmed.ncbi.nlm.nih.gov/25752756/

8. NIH Consensus Development Program Archive. "Implications of Obesity. Consensus Development Conference Statement." U.S. Department of Health and Human Services: National Institute of Health.

February 11-13, 1985. https://consensus.nih.gov/1985/1985Obesity-049html.htm

CHAPTER TWO

1. Ashlee Bennett. Quote from Instagram account, Bodyimage_therapist. Published March 11, 2021. https://www.instagram.com/bodyimage_therapist.
2. Kathleen M. Rasmussen, P.M. Catalano, and A.L. Yaktine. "New Guidelines for Weight Gain During Pregnancy: What Obstetrician/Gynecologists Should Know." Current Opinion in Obstetrics & Gynecology 21, no. 6 (2009): 521–526. https://doi.org/10.1097/GCO.0b013e-328332d24e
3. Angela C. Incollingo Rodriguez, C. Dunkel Schetter, A. Brewis, and A.J. Tomiyama. "The Psychological Burden of Baby Weight: Pregnancy, Weight Stigma, and Maternal Health." Social Science & Medicine, no 235 (2019). https://www.sciencedirect.com/science/article/abs/pii/S0277953619303879
4. Ewelina Rogozińska, J. Zamora, N. Marlin, A. Pilar Betran, A. Astrup, A. Bogaerts, J.G. Cecatti, J.M. Dodd, F. Facchinetti., N.R.W. Geiker, et al. "Gestational Weight Gain Outside the Institute of Medicine Recommendations and Adverse Pregnancy Outcomes: Analysis Using Individual Participant Data from Randomised Trials." BMC Pregnancy Childbirth 19, no. 322 (2019). https://doi.org/10.1186/s12884-019-2472-7
5. Connie L. Bish, S.Y. Chu, C.K. Shapiro-Mendoza, A.J. Sharma, and H.M. Blanck. "Trying to Lose or Maintain Weight During Pregnancy-United States, 2003." Maternal Child Health Journal 13, no. 2 (2009): 286-292. https://pubmed.ncbi.nlm.nih.gov/18449630/
6. Stephanie Dodier. "Body Neutrality." The Beyond the Food Show. Podcast audio. September 24, 2020.
7. Laura Thomas, Just Eat It: How Intuitive Eating Can Help You Get Your Shit Together Around Food. London: Blue Books, 2019, 13-16.
8. Evelyn Tribole and Elyse Resch, Intuitive Eating: a Revolutionary Program that Works. New York: St. Martin's Press, 2012, 281-297.
9. Laura Grady. "Women are calling out Instagram for censoring photos of fat bodies." Flare. October 18, 2018. https://www.flare.com/news/instagram-censorship-fat-plus-size/
10. Makeda Loney, J. Oliver, and M. Smith. "Digital Decapitation." Fat Outta Hell. Podcast audio. August 26 2020.
11. Mia O'Malley. "My Invisible Plus Size Pregnancy" Plus Size Birth Blog. Accessed March 11, 2021. https://plussizebirth.com/my-invisible-plus-size-pregnancy/
12. Elena R. Magro☐Malosso, G. Saccone, M. Di Tommaso, A. Roman,

and V. Berghella. "Exercise During Pregnancy and Risk of Gestational Hypertensive Disorders: a Systematic Review and Meta□analysis." Acta Obstetricia et Gynecologica Scandinavica 96, no. 8 (2017): 921– 931. https://pubmed.ncbi.nlm.nih.gov/28401531/

13. Cuilin Zhang, C.G. Solomon, J.E. Manson, and F.B. Hu. "A Prospective Study of Pregravid Physical Activity and Sedentary Behaviors in Relation to the Risk for Gestational Diabetes Mellitus." Archives of Internal Medicine 166, no. 5 (2006): 543-548. https://pubmed.ncbi.nlm.nih.gov/16534041/

14. Gaston Anca and H. Prapavessis. "Tired, Moody and Pregnant? Exercise May be the Answer." Psychology & Health 28, no. 12 (2013): 1353-1369. https://pubmed.ncbi.nlm.nih.gov/23837826/

15. Marcelo C. de Barros, M.A. Lopes, R.P. Francisco, A.D. Sapienza, and M. Zugaib. "Resistance Exercise and Glycemic Control in Women with Gestational Diabetes Mellitus." American Journal of Obstetrics and Gynecology 203, no. 6 (2010): 556. https://pubmed.ncbi.nlm.nih.gov/20864072/

16. Ruben Barakat, M. Pelaez, C. Lopez, R. Montejo, and J. Coteron. "Exercise During Pregnancy Reduces the Rate of Cesarean and Instrumental Deliveries: Results of a Randomized Controlled Trial." The Journal Maternal-Fetal Neonatal Medicine 25, no. 11 (2012): 2372-2376. https://pubmed.ncbi.nlm.nih.gov/22715981/

17. Kristin R. Kardel, B. Johansen, N. Voldner, P.O. Iversen, and T. Henriksen. "Association Between Aerobic Fitness in Late Pregnancy and Duration of Labor in Nulliparous Women." Acta Obstetricia et Gynecologica Scandinavica 88, no. 8 (2009): 948-952. https://pubmed.ncbi.nlm.nih.gov/19562561/

18. MissFits Workout®website: https://www.missfitsworkout.co.uk/

CHAPTER THREE

1. Elaine Zwelling. "The Emergence of High-tech Birthing." Journal of Obstetric, Gynecologic and Neonatal Nursing 37, no. 1 (2008): 85-93. https://www.jognn.org/article/S0884-2175(15)33713-8/fulltext

2. Richard Johanson, M. Newburn, and A. Macfarlane. "Has the Medicalisation of Childbirth Gone Too Far?" BMJ 324, no. 7342 (2002): 892–895. https://pubmed.ncbi.nlm.nih.gov/11950741/

3. Peter M. Dunn. "The Chamberlen Family (1560–1728) and Obstetric Forceps," Archives of Disease in Childhood - Fetal and Neonatal Edition 81, no. 3 (1999): F232-F235. https://fn.bmj.com/content/81/3/F232

4. Karla Papagni and E. Buckner. "Doula Support and Attitudes of Intrapartum Nurses: A Qualitative Study from the Patient's Perspective."

The Journal of Perinatal Education 15, no. 1 (2006): 11–18. https://doi.org/10.1624/105812406X92949

5. Maire O Regan. "Active Management of Labour: the Irish Way of Birth." AIMS Journal 10, no. 2 (1998): 1-10. https://www.aims.org.uk/pdfs/journal/6

6. Olufemi T. Oladapo, J.P. Souza, B. Fawole, K. Mugerwa, G. Perdoná, D. Alves, H. Souza, R. Reis, L. Oliveira-Ciabati, A. Maiorano, et al. "Progression of the First Stage of Spontaneous Labour: A Prospective Cohort Study in Two Sub-Saharan African Countries." PLoS Medicine 15, no. 1 (2018). https://www.ncbi.nlm.nih.gov/pmc/articles/PMC5770022/

7. Shayna M. Norman, M.G. Tuuli, A.O. Odibo, A.B. Caughey, K.A. Roehl, and A.G. Cahill. "The Effects of Obesity on the First Stage of Labor." Obstetrics and Gynecology 120, no. 1 (2012): 130–135. https://pubmed.ncbi.nlm.nih.gov/22914401/

8. Fay Menacker and B.E. Hamilton. "Recent Trends in Cesarean Delivery in the United States." NCHS Data Brief, no. 35 (2010): 1-8. https://pubmed.ncbi.nlm.nih.gov/20334736/

9. Jacqui Wise. "Alarming Global Rise in Caesarean Births, Figures Show." BMJ 363, (2018). https://www.bmj.com/content/363/bmj.k4319

10. Hollie Ewers. "Proportion of induced labours rise" Royal College of Midwives. October 26, 2018. https://www.rcm.org.uk/news-views/news/proportion-of-induced-labours-rise/

11. Eugene R . Declercq, C. Sakala, M.P. Corry, S. Applebaum, and A. Herrlich. Listening to Mothers SM III: Pregnancy and Birth. New York: Childbirth Connection, May 2013.

12. David P. Johnson, N.R. Davis, and A.J. Brown. "Risk of Cesarean Delivery After Induction at Term in Nulliparous Women with an Unfavorable Cervix." American Journal of Obstetrics and Gynecology 188, no. 6 (2003): 1569-1572. https://pubmed.ncbi.nlm.nih.gov/12824994/

13. Karen Louise Ellekjaer, T. Bergholt and E. Løkkegaard. "Maternal Obesity and Its Effect on Labour Duration in Nulliparous Women: a Retrospective Observational Cohort Study. BMC Pregnancy Childbirth 17, no. 222 (2017). https://doi.org/10.1186/s12884-017-1413-6

14. Joyce A Martin, B.E. Hamilton, P.D. Sutton, S.J. Ventura, F. Menacker, and M.L. Munson. "Births: Final Data for 2002." National Vital Statistics Reports 52, no. 10 (2003): 1-113. https://pubmed.ncbi.nlm.nih.gov/14717305/

15. Lisa Heelan. "Fetal Monitoring: Creating a Culture of Safety with Informed Choice." The Journal of Perinatal Education 22, no. 3 (2013): 156–165. https://doi.org/10.1891/1058-1243.22.3.156

16. Zarko Alfirevic, D. Devane, and G.M. Gyte. "Continuous Cardiotocography (CTG) as a Form of Electronic Fetal Monitoring (EFM) for Fetal Assessment During Labour." The Cochrane Database of

Systematic Reviews 19, no. 3 (2006). https://pubmed.ncbi.nlm.nih. gov/16856111/

17. Thomas P. Sartwelle and J.C. Johnston. "Continuous Electronic Fetal Monitoring During Labor: A Critique and a Reply to Contemporary Proponents." Surgery Journal 4, no. 1 (2018). https://pubmed.ncbi. nlm.nih.gov/29527573/

18. Paul Lewis. "Room 101 – The Only Place for Fetal Monitoring in Labour." British Journal of Midwifery 21, no. 6 (2013): 386.

19. Thomas P. Sartwelle and J.C. Johnston. "Cerebral Palsy Litigation: Change Course or Abandon Ship." Journal of Child Neurology 30, no. 7 (2015). https://pubmed.ncbi.nlm.nih.gov/25183322/

20. Karin B. Nelson, T.P. Sartwelle and D.J. Rouse. (2016). "Electronic Fetal Monitoring, Cerebral palsy, and Caesarean Section: Assumptions Versus Evidence." BMJ (Clinical Research ed.) 355, (2016). https://www.ncbi.nlm.nih.gov/pmc/articles/PMC6883481/

21. Suellen Miller, A. Edgardo, M. Chamillard, A. Ciapponi, D. Colaci, D. Comandé, V. Diaz, S. Geller, C. Hanson, A. Langer, et al. "Beyond Too Little, Too Late and Too Much, Too Soon: a Pathway Towards Evidence-Based, Respectful Maternity Care Worldwide," The Lancet 388, no. 10056 (2016): 2176-2192. https://doi.org/10.1016/S0140-6736(16)31472-6

22. Amy Dockser. "To Reduce C-Sections, Change the Culture of the Labor Ward." The Wall Street Journal. Sept 12, 2017. https://www. wsj.com/articles/to-reduce-c-sections-change-the-culture-of-the-labor-ward-1505268661

CHAPTER FOUR

1. Soo M. Downe, K. Finlayson, Ö. Tunçalp, and A. Metin Gülmezoglu. "What Matters to Women: a Systematic Scoping Review to Identify the Processes and Outcomes of Antenatal Care Provision That Are Important to Healthy Pregnant Women." BJOG 123, no 4 (2016): 529– 539. https://pubmed.ncbi.nlm.nih.gov/26701735/

2. Soo M. Downe, K. Dinlayson, O.T. Oladapo, M. Bonet and A.M. Gülmezoglu. "What Matters to Women During Childbirth: A systematic Qualitative Review." PloS one 13, no. 4 (2018). https://doi. org/10.1371/journal.pone.0194906

3. Jane Sandall, H. Soltani, S. Gates, A. Shennan, and D. Devane. "Midwife□led Continuity Models Versus Other Models of Care for Childbearing Women." Cochrane Database of Systematic Reviews, no. 4 (2016). https://www.cochranelibrary.com/cdsr/ doi/10.1002/14651858.CD004667.pub5/full

4. Egle Bartuseviciene, J. Kacerauskiene, A. Bartuseviciu, M. Pauliony-te, R.J. Nadisauskiene, M. Kliucinskas, V. Stankeviciute, L. Maleck-

iene, and D.R. Railaite. "Comparison of Midwife-led and Obstetrician-led Care in Lithuania: A retrospective Cohort Study." Midwifery, (2018): 67-71. https://pubmed.ncbi.nlm.nih.gov/29980361/.

5. Cecelia M. Jevitt, S. Stapleton, Y. Deng, X. Song, K. Wang, and D.R. Jolles. "Birth Outcomes of Women with Obesity Enrolled for Care at Freestanding Birth Centers in the United States." Journal of Midwifery & Women's Health 66, no. 1 (2021): 14-23. https://doi.org/10.1111/jmwh.13194.

6. "Perinatal and Maternal Outcomes by Planned Place of Birth for Healthy Women with Low Risk Pregnancies: the Birthplace in England National Prospective Cohort Study." BMJ 343, (2011). https://www.bmj.com/content/343/bmj.d7400.

7. Angela C. Incollingo Rodriguez, C. Dunkel Schetter, A. Brewis, and A.J. Tomiyama. "The Psychological Burden of Baby Weight: Pregnancy, Weight Stigma, and Maternal Health." Social Science & Medicine, no 235 (2019). https://www.sciencedirect.com/science/article/abs/pii/S0277953619303879

8. Charlotte A De Vries and RG De Vries. "Childbirth Education in the 21st Century: an Immodest Proposal." The Journal of Perinatal Education 16, no. 4 (2007): 38–48. https://doi.org/10.1624/105812407X244958

9. "Why take classes in The Bradley Method® of natural childbirth?" Bradley Birth. March 18, 2021. http://bradleybirth.com/WhyBradley.aspx

10. "The Lamaze Difference." Lamaze International. March 18, 2021. https://www.lamaze.org/parenting-practices

11. Azzahra Badaruddin Fatimah. "Birth Preparations: Impacts on the Birthing Outcomes." Final year research project, University College Cork, Ireland, 2017.

12. Debs Neiger. Quote from Instagram account, Debsagos. Published March 13, 2021. www.instagram.com/debsagos

13. Jennifer Fenwick, J. Toohill, J. Gamble, D.K. Creedy, A. Buist, E. Turkstra, A. Sneddon, P.A. Scuffham and E. Ryding. "Effects of a Midwife Psycho-Education Intervention to Reduce Childbirth Fear on Women's Birth Outcomes and Postpartum Psychological Wellbeing." BMC Pregnancy Childbirth 15, 284 (2015). https://doi.org/10.1186/s12884-015-0721-y

14. Hanna Rouhe, K. Salmela□Aro, R. Toivanen, M. Tokola, E. Halmesmäki, and T. Saisto. "Obstetric Outcome After Intervention for Severe Fear of Childbirth in Nulliparous Women – Randomised Trial." BJOG: An International Journal of Obstetrics & Gynaecology 120, no. 1 (2013): 75-84. https://doi.org/10.1111/1471-0528.12011

15. Siw Alehagen, K. Wijma, and B. Wijma. "Fear During Labor." Acta Obstetricia et Gynecologica Scandinavica 80, no. 4 (2001): 315-320. https://doi.org/10.1034/j.1600-0412.2001.080004315.x

16. Robab Hassanzadeh, F. Abbas-Alizadeh, S. Meedya, S. Mo-hammad-Alizadeh-Charandabi, and M. Mirghafourvand. "Fear of Childbirth, Anxiety and Depression in Three Groups of Primiparous Pregnant Women Not Attending, Irregularly Attending and Regularly Attending Childbirth Preparation Classes." BMC Women's Health 20, no. 180 (2020). https://doi.org/10.1186/s12905-020-01048-9

17. Robab Hassanzadeh, F. Abbas-Alizadeh, S. Meedya, S. Moham-mad-Alizadeh-Charandabi, and M. Mirghafourvand. "Comparison of Childbirth Experiences and Postpartum Depression Among Prim-iparous Women Based on Their Attendance in Childbirth Prepara-tion Classes." The Journal of Maternal-Fetal & Neonatal Medicine, (2020): 1-8. https://pubmed.ncbi.nlm.nih.gov/33076724/

18. Larissa G. Duncan, M.A. Cohn, M.T. Chao, J.G. Cook, J. Riccobono and N. Bardacke. "Benefits of Preparing for Childbirth with Mind-fulness Training: a Randomized Controlled Trial with Active Com-parison." BMC Pregnancy Childbirth 17, no. 1 (2017): 140. https://pubmed.ncbi.nlm.nih.gov/28499376/

CHAPTER FIVE

1. "Birth Survey 2016" Positive Birth Movement. March 24, 2019. https://www.positivebirthmovement.org/birth-survey-2016/

2. Hanna Dahlen. "Don't throw the birth plan out with the bath water!" The Ethics Centre Blog. August 2, 2016. https://ethics.org.au/dont-throw-the-birth-plan-out-with-the-birth-water/

3. Mary Regan and J. Liaschenko. "In the Mind of the Beholder: Hy-pothesized Effect of Intrapartum Nurses' Cognitive Frames of Child-birth Cesarean Section Rates." Qualitative Health Research 17, no. 5 (2007): 612-624. https://experts.umn.edu/en/publications/in-the-mind-of-the-beholder-hypothesized-effect-of-intrapartum-nu

4. Stephan Oelhafen, M. Trachsel, S. Monteverde, L. Raio and E. Cignacco Müller. "Informal Coercion During Childbirth: Risk Factors and Prevalence Estimates from a Nationwide Survey Among Women in Switzerland." BMC Pregnancy Childbirth 21, no. 1 (2021). https://pubmed.ncbi.nlm.nih.gov/33971841/

5. Helen Stapleton, M. Kirkham, and G. Thomas. "Qualitative Study of Evidence Based Leaflets in Maternity Care." BMJ Clinical Re-search ed. 324, no. 7338 (2002): 639. https://pubmed.ncbi.nlm.nih.gov/11895821/

6. Sara Wickham. "The language of the complicated." Dr Sara Wick-ham. December 10, 2018. https://www.sarawickham.com/articles-2/the-language-of-the-complicated/

7. Sara Wickham."Word-thought for the day: replacing risk with chance." Dr Sara Wickham. November 26, 2018. https://www.

sarawickham.com/quotes-and-shares/word-thought-for-the-day-re-placing-risk-with-choice/

8. "Working Together to Reduce Black Maternal Mortality." Centers for Disease Control and Prevention. April 9, 2021 https://www.cdc.gov/healthequity/features/maternal-mortality/index.html

9. Kate E. Marti, R.M. Grivell, L.N. Yelland and J.M. Dodd. "The Influence of Maternal BMI and Gestational Diabetes on Pregnancy Outcome." Diabetes Research and Clinical Practice 108, no. 3 (2015): 508-513. https://pubmed.ncbi.nlm.nih.gov/25796512/

10. Elizabeth R. Moore, G.C. Anderson, N. Bergman, and T. Dowswell. "Early Skin-to-Skin Contact for Mothers and Their Healthy Newborn Infants." The Cochrane Database of Systematic Reviews 5, no. 5 (2012). https://doi.org/10.1002/14651858.CD003519.pub3

11. Monash University. "Skin-to-skin 'kangaroo care' shows important benefits for premature babies." Science Daily. May 7, 2020. www.sciencedaily.com/releases/2020/05/200507102434.htm

12. Boulvain Michel, C Stan, and O Irion. "Membrane Sweeping for Induction of Labour." The Cochrane Database Systematic Reviews (2005). https://www.cochranelibrary.com/cdsr/doi/10.1002/14651858.CD000451.pub2/full

13. Jessica Hanae Zafra-Tanaka, R. Montesinos-Segura, P. Flores-Gonzales, and A. Taype-Rondan. "Potential Excess of Vaginal Examinations During the Management of Labor: Frequency and Associated Factors in 13 Peruvian Hospitals." Reproductive Health 16, no. 146 (2019). https://doi.org/10.1186/s12978-019-0811-9

14. Siew Fan Wong, S.K. Hui, H. Choi and L.C. Ho. "Does Sweeping of Membranes Beyond 40 Weeks Reduce the Need for Formal Induction of Labour? BJOG 109, no. 6 (2002): 632-636. https://pubmed.ncbi.nlm.nih.gov/12118640/

15. Micah J Hill, G.D. McWilliams, D. Garcia-Sur, B. Chen, M. Munroe, and N.J. Hoeldtke. "The Effect of Membrane Sweeping on Prelabor Rupture of Membranes: a Randomized Controlled Trial." Obstetrics and Gynecology 11, no. 6 (2008): 1313-1319. https://pubmed.ncbi.nlm.nih.gov/18515514/

16. Max Mongelli, M. Wilcox, and J. Gardosi. "Estimating the Date of Confinement: Ultrasonographic Biometry Versus Certain Menstrual Dates." American Journal of Obstetrics and Gynecology 174, no 1 (1996): 278-281. https://pubmed.ncbi.nlm.nih.gov/8572021/

17. Sarah J Buckley. "Executive Summary. In Hormonal Physiology of Childbearing: Evidence and Implications for Women, Babies, and Maternity Care." The Journal of Perinatal Education 24, no. 3 (2015): 145-153. https://www.ncbi.nlm.nih.gov/pmc/articles/PMC4720867/

CHAPTER SIX

1. Meghan A Bohren, G.J. Hofmeyr, C. Sakala, R.K. Fukuzawa, and A. Cuthbert. "Continuous Support for Women During Childbirth." Cochrane Database of Systematic Reviews 7, no. 7 (2017). https://pubmed.ncbi.nlm.nih.gov/28681500/
2. Sarah J. Buckley. "Executive Summary. In Hormonal Physiology of Childbearing: Evidence and Implications for Women, Babies, and Maternity Care." The Journal of Perinatal Education 24, no. 3 (2015): 145-153. https://www.ncbi.nlm.nih.gov/pmc/articles/PMC4720867/
3. Anita J Gagnon and K. Waghorn. "Supportive Care by Maternity Nurses: a Work Sampling Study in an Intrapartum Unit." Birth 23, no. 1 (1996): 1-6. https://pubmed.ncbi.nlm.nih.gov/8703251/
4. Ramin Ravangard, A. Basiri, Z. Sajjadnia, and N. Shokrpour. "Comparison of the Effects of Using Physiological Methods and Accompanying a Doula in Deliveries on Nulliparous Women's Anxiety and Pain: A Case Study in Iran." The Health Care Manager 36, no. 4 (2017): 372-379. https://pubmed.ncbi.nlm.nih.gov/28961642/
5. "Safe Prevention of the Primary Cesarean Delivery." Obstetric Care Consensus No. 1. American College of Obstetricians and Gynecologists. (2014): 693-711. https://www.acog.org/clinical/clinical-guidance/obstetric-care-consensus/articles/2014/03/safe-prevention-of-the-primary-cesarean-delivery#

About the Author

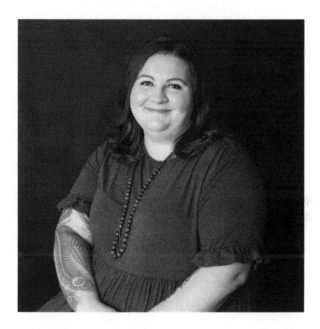

Michelle is a certified birth and postpartum doula, childbirth educator and hypnobirthing teacher. She has made it her mission to change the way people approach fat pregnancy and birth. Through her teaching and social media networks, she seeks to empower and educate plus size expecting parents— and their birth partners— so they may seek the positive birth they want and deserve.